CONCISE GUIDE TO
Neuropsychiatry and Behavioral Neurology

D0250798

American Psychiatric Press
CONCISE GUIDES

Robert E. Hales, M.D.
Series Editor

CONCISE GUIDE TO
Neuropsychiatry and Behavioral Neurology

Jeffrey L. Cummings, M.D.
Professor of Neurology and Psychiatry &
Biobehavioral Science
UCLA School of Medicine
Chief, Behavioral Neuroscience Section
Psychiatry Service
West Los Angeles Veterans Affairs
Medical Center
Los Angeles, California

Michael R. Trimble, M.D., F.R.C.P., F.R.C.Psych.
Professor of Behavioural Neurology
Institute of Neurology
Queen Square
London, England

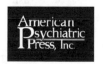

Washington, DC
London, England

Copyright © 1995 American Psychiatric Press, Inc.
ALL RIGHTS RESERVED
Manufactured in the United States of America on acid-free paper
98   97   96   95   4   3   2   1
First Edition

American Psychiatric Press, Inc.
1400 K Street, N.W., Washington, DC   20005

Library of Congress Cataloging-in-Publication Data
Cummings, Jeffrey L., 1948–
    Concise guide to neuropsychiatry and behavioral neurology /
Jeffrey L. Cummings, Michael R. Trimble.
        p.   cm.
    Includes bibliographical references and index.
    ISBN 0-88048-493-4 (alk. paper)
    1. Neurobehavioral disorders.   2. Neuropsychiatry.   I.
Trimble, Michael R.   II. Title.
    [DNLM: 1. Brain Diseases—physiopathology.   2. Mental
Disorders—diagnosis.   3. Mental Disorders—therapy.
4. Neuropsychology.   WL 348 C971c 1995]
RC386.C86   1995
616.8—dc20
DNLM/DLC
for Library of Congress   95-1386
                                                                CIP

British Library Cataloguing in Publication Data
A CIP record is available from the British Library.

This volume is dedicated to

D. Frank Benson, M.D.,

who guided our interest in neuropsychiatry,
and to all the students who find this small book
sufficiently tantalizing to pursue their own interests
in neuropsychiatry.

CONTENTS

TABLES

FIGURES

INTRODUCTION

to the American Psychiatric Press Concise Guides

The *American Psychiatric Press Concise Guides* series provides practical information for psychiatrists, psychiatry residents, and medical students working in a variety of treatment settings, such as inpatient psychiatry units, outpatient clinics, consultation-liaison services, or private office settings. The *Concise Guides* are meant to complement more detailed information found in lengthier psychiatry texts.

The *Concise Guides* address topics of greatest concern to psychiatrists in clinical practice. The books in this series contain a detailed table of contents, along with an index, tables, and charts for easy access. The books are designed to fit into a coat pocket, which makes them a convenient source of information. The number of references has been limited to those most relevant to the material presented.

For neuropsychiatrists, behavioral neurologists, and psychiatrists who are interested in evaluating and treating patients with both neurological and psychiatric disorders, the *Concise Guide to Neuropsychiatry and Behavioral Neurology,* by Jeffrey L. Cummings, M.D., and Michael R. Trimble, M.D., F.R.C.P., F.R.C.Psych., provides an outstanding overview of this rapidly changing specialty area.

One unique characteristic of this Concise Guide is that it is the first one written by authors from the United States and England, with Dr. Cummings at the University of California, Los Angeles, and Dr. Trimble at the Institute of Neurology, Queen Square, London. Each author is an outstanding educator, clinician, and scientist.

Because a high percentage of patients with neurological disorders (such as dementia, Parkinson's disease, traumatic brain injury, and many others) exhibit psychiatric symptoms or disorders, this *Concise Guide* is of significant value to psychiatrists and neurologists working in general hospital settings, psychiatry and neurology residents, and medical students who may rotate on a psychiatry consultation service. It complements the existing major texts in the field; in particular, *Behavioral Neurology,* coauthored by Gary J. Tucker, M.D., and Jonathan Pincus, M.D.; *Clinical Neuropsychiatry,* edited by Jeffrey L. Cummings, M.D.; and *The American Psychiatric Press Textbook of Neuropsychiatry,* Second Edition, edited by Stuart C. Yudofsky, M.D., and me. The reader is encouraged to turn to these more extensive texts for more complete information.

Cummings and Trimble begin this *Concise Guide* by providing an overview of the neuropsychiatric assessment, focusing in particular on the clinical and laboratory examination of the patient. They then turn to behavioral neurobiology and provide a review of important neurophysiological and neurochemical concepts. Next is a summary of major neuroanatomical landmarks, with an emphasis on the limbic system, the basal ganglia, and the reticular activating system. The authors provide an overview of neuropsychiatric symptoms and syndromes, with a focus on depression, mania, mood lability, psychosis, hallucinations, anxiety, obsessive-compulsive disorder, personality changes, dissociative disorders, and altered sexual behavior.

Cummings and Trimble also summarize a host of specific neurological syndromes and dysfunctions. They discuss in a complete yet concise manner frontal lobe syndromes, aphasia and related syndromes, visual and visual-spatial disorders, memory disturbances, epilepsy and the limbic system, dementia and delirium, movement disorders, stroke, white matter diseases, errors of metabolism, and head injury. They end the book with a discussion of treatments in neuropsychiatry with a focus on the major neuropsychiatric medications: antidepressants, major tranquilizers, minor tranquilizers, mood-stabilizing drugs, and anticonvulsant medications. They also provide a brief summary of electroconvulsive therapy and neurosurgical procedures.

The chapters are very well written and contain many clinical pearls. In addition, the authors have included many excellent figures and tables that summarize important clinical information in an abbreviated fashion. Psychiatrists and neurologists, and especially residents in both specialties, should find this pocket-size guide essential and carry it with them in their laboratory coat, along with their stethoscope and reflex hammer.

The authors have done an outstanding job in summarizing the most important syndromes and concepts in the field of neuropsychiatry and behavioral neurology. The *Concise Guide to Neuropsychiatry and Behavioral Neurology* also complements quite nicely the recently published *Concise Guide to Consultation Psychiatry,* Second Edition, by Michael G. Wise, M.D., and James R. Rundell, M.D. Wise and Rundell focus more on the diagnosis and treatment of disorders in medically ill patients, whereas Cummings and Trimble examine patients more from a combined neurological and psychiatric perspective.

In summary, I have found myself reading this book again and again and learning more each time. Readers should be very pleased with their purchase of this latest addition to the *Concise Guides* series.

Robert E. Hales, M.D.
Series Editor
American Psychiatric Press Concise Guides Series

PREFACE

Neuropsychiatry and behavioral neurology are evolving disciplines devoted to understanding the behavioral consequences of brain dysfunction and to using this information to improve patient care. Neuropsychiatry emphasizes psychiatric disorders associated with brain dysfunction such as poststroke depression and epilepsy-related psychosis, whereas behavioral neurology addresses deficit syndromes such as aphasia, amnesia, and agnosia. Both these approaches are critical to fully assessing and managing patients with brain disorders.

The current volume provides brief synopses of the major neuropsychiatric and neurobehavioral syndromes, discusses their clinical assessment, and provides guidelines for management. The volume is intended to provide the most critical facts, plus bibliographies that guide more extensive reading. This is a reference text that can be used to quickly access diagnostic and treatment information. To achieve the intended brevity, we eschewed exhaustive reviews of the available literature and chose to provide focused summaries of the clinical features, underlying pathophysiology, and treatment options for the major neuropsychiatric disorders.

Neuropsychiatry and behavioral neurology are rapidly growing disciplines. This growth is driven by four forces: 1) the aging of the population with the attendant marked increase in age-related neuropsychiatric morbidity associated with dementia, stroke, and Parkinson's disease; 2) rapid improvement in neuroimaging techniques that allow the visualization of many dimensions of brain function and anatomic structure—including glucose metabolism, blood flow, dopamine distribution, and serotonin receptors—that are related to behavioral changes; 3) emergence of new therapies that change brain function to effect a behavioral change, including serotonin uptake blockers for obsessive-compulsive disorder and depression, cholinesterase inhibitors for Alzheimer's disease, GABAergic anticonvulsants, and neuroprotective agents for degenerative disorders; and 4) marked growth of the neurosciences with potential applicability to understanding the neurobiologic basis of human behavior, including the development of animal models of several disorders, discovery of the genetic etiology of many diseases, and revelation through molecular biologic techniques of the cascade of events that transform genetic changes into cellular alterations and eventually into behavioral manifestations. We furnish the current clinically applicable conclusions of this enormous body of work. Our aim is to provide a distillate that can be used in the course of clinical care.

We hope that this small volume helps practitioners to provide the most up-to-date care to their patients and that it stimulates the interest of students and practicing physicians in this exciting field.

NEUROPSYCHIATRIC ASSESSMENT

Neuropsychiatry and behavioral neurology are clinical disciplines devoted to understanding and treating behavioral disturbances associated with brain dysfunction. Detection and characterization of brain disorders require a careful clinical assessment as well as the application of selected neurodiagnostic procedures. In this chapter we discuss clinical examination as well as neuropsychological testing, laboratory tests, electrophysiologic techniques, and brain imaging. The symptoms of brain dysfunction are presented in more detail in Chapter 3, and the symptoms of each specific disease or condition are presented in the relevant chapters of the book.

■ DEFINITIONS

Symptoms are the complaints of the patient that are spontaneously reported or elicited by the clinical history. *Signs* are observed by the physician, the patient, or the patient's friends or relatives and indicate the presence of abnormal functioning of one or more body systems.

A *syndrome* is a constellation of signs and symptoms that seem to coalesce to provide a recognizable entity with its defining characteristics. Syndromes may be classified, and they are the clinical representatives of illness. The latter is what the patient presents to the physician with, which in part may represent the expression of disease. However, the presentation of an illness depends on many factors, including environmental and personality variables.

■ CLINICAL AND LABORATORY EXAMINATION

INITIAL OBSERVATIONS

First observe, and then listen. The patient's dress may reveal the eccentricity of hysteria or the flamboyance of mania or may hint at the dishevelment of schizophrenia or dementia. Is eye contact maintained? The posture may be that of the universally flexed melancholic or parkinsonian patient, or it may be the stilted stance of a schizophrenic person.

Disturbances of motor activity may aid diagnosis. In *catatonia,* muscle tone is high, leading to resistance, and in *flexibilitas cerea (catalepsy),* limbs and postures can be maintained for hours at a time. *Gegenhalten* refers to the finding that passive resistance to movement of a limb increases in direct relation to the force that is applied by the examiner.

The gait may suggest extrapyramidal disorder, with smaller steps and poverty of accessory movements in parkinsonism. *Akinesia,* with poverty of movement, is seen in patients receiving neuroleptic treatment. The patient with *akathisia* may not be able to sit for longer than a few minutes. The patient with agitation paces. *Mannerisms* (exaggerated components of the usual behavioral repertoire), *stereotypies* (repeated complex sequences of purposeless movement), and *choreoathetoid* writhing may be noted. Mannerisms and stereotypies are common in schizophrenia; choreoathetoid writhing may suggest any number of extrapyramidal problems. *Tics* (which are frequent stereotyped repetitive movements of small groups of muscles) may suggest Tourette syndrome. Vocal tics and excessive sniffing or clearing of the throat are also characteristic of this disorder.

The mouth may writhe, as in *tardive dyskinesia,* or form more sustained abnormal postures, as in a *dystonia.* The lips may reveal the lesions of vitamin deficiency, the scars of self-mutilation, or the dryness of anxiety.

The hands may tremble in cases of anxiety or extrapyramidal disease. Is there any evidence of muscle wasting (loss of muscle bulk generally or in specific areas)? The fingers may reveal nicotine addiction, and bitten nails may suggest an anxiety neurosis. On shaking the patient's hand, the clinician may detect the clammy sweat of anxiety or an underlying extrapyramidal tremor. Handshaking also gives the opportunity to test for a grasp reflex. Left-handedness should be noted, as it may suggest reorganization of cerebral function consequent to early cerebral damage.

The patient's speech is studied for form and content. The slowing of depression contrasts with the pressured overactivity of mania. *Dysarthria,* due to impairment of the neuromuscular mechanisms of speech, may hint at intoxication or cerebral or cerebellar damage. A stammer reveals anxiety; paraphasias and neologisms indicate aphasia or schizophrenia. Attention and concentration, the ability to maintain a stream of thought, and the ability to converse should be noted.

The *prosody* of speech refers to its melodic intonation. It may be flat in cases of schizophrenia or after right-hemisphere lesions.

Formal thought disorder, which refers to disorganization and concretization of thought processes, suggests either schizophrenia or a neurologic disease. Slowing of the train of thought is seen with the psychomotor slowing of depression and with the bradyphrenia of many neurologic disorders such as head injury, Parkinson's disease, epilepsy, and multiple sclerosis. *Viscosity* describes the "sticky thinking" of some such patients. *Circumstantiality* refers to a persistent tendency to wander slowly over the irrelevant details of a subject before reaching a final conclusion.

Delusions are unshakable beliefs that are manifestly incorrect, even when the patient's cultural surrounding is taken into account. *Autochthonous delusions* arise suddenly, fully formed and spontaneously. They are bizarre and nearly always signify schizophrenia. *Hallucinations* are percepts without objects, and *illusions* are abnormal perceptions of sensory stimuli. Does the patient have insight into his or her medical and mental state?

Hyperesthesia, especially for sounds, is not uncommon in anxious patients; *hypoesthesia* is frequent in depression. Anesthesia, in the sense of reporting *anesthetic patches* or *hemianesthesia* may be seen in patients with hysteria (conversion disorder).

Alterations in size of objects such as micropsia and macropsia may suggest ophthalmological disease or temporal lobe dysfunction. *Derealization* and *depersonalization,* in which the world and the patients themselves, respectively, feel different, unreal, empty, or two-dimensional, are noted in a variety of conditions but especially in anxiety and as an aura in temporal lobe epilepsy. In *déjà vu* experiences, patients feel that everything they are experiencing has happened before. *Jamais vu* is the opposite, an abnormal feeling of unfamiliarity.

Careful attention should be paid to the patient's mood and to whether delusions are congruent or incongruent to the mood state. Mood-incongruent delusions immediately hint at schizophrenia. Apathy is common after cerebral damage, but it is seen in a wide range of neuropsychiatric disorders. *Emotional lability* is noted when the patient is unable to control his or her emotional flow, laughing at the hint of a joke or crying at the hint of sadness. *Pseudobulbar palsy* is a common form of emotional lability. It is contrasted with the empty euphoria of patients with multiple sclerosis, and the meaningless, playful *witzelsucht* of frontal lobe dysfunction. Inappropriate affect is more characteristic of schizophrenia.

NEUROPSYCHOLOGICAL TESTING

Although formal testing is done in the laboratory, clinical mental status testing can be very valuable, and in many patients it is an essential part of the initial screening. This clinical testing is outlined in Table 1–1. These tests should be done routinely, but any suspicion of higher cognitive dysfunction should lead to a request for more formal testing. It is necessary to specify the kind of deficit anticipated—for example, to ask that attention be paid to tests of frontal lobe function.

Patients with confusional states cannot be reliably tested, but the degree, content, and variability of their mental state must be noted. Patients with typical *delirium* seem confused and are disoriented for time and possibly also for place. Simple mental arithmetic is poorly performed, and memory is unreliable. Hallucinations are predominantly visual, complex, and silent. Delusions are often paranoid. Typically, the severity of the symptoms fluctuates with time.

Attention can be tested by repetition of digits or by the serial 7s (or serial 3s) subtraction test. Longer periods of attention *(vigi-*

TABLE 1–1. **Bedside mental state testing**

Assess level of consciousness

Observe and assess orientation for time, place, and person

Assess attention and vigilance

    Digit repetition

    Serial 7 subtraction

    Digit reversal

    Days or months in reverse order

Test verbal output

    Rate, rhythm, syntax, and semantics

    Speech errors

Ask patient to point to objects in the environment named by the examiner

Ask patient to perform simple commands

Ask patient to name objects, body parts, and colors

Ask patient to

    Read a passage of simple text (e.g., from a newspaper) and test comprehension

    Write his or her name and a short paragraph on a subject of interest to him or her

Test memory ability

    Repeat the Babcock sentence ("The one thing a nation needs in order to be rich and great is a large secure supply of wood," or "The clouds hung low in the valley and the wind howled among the trees as the men went on through the rain")

    Repeat a story

    Remember four words

    Test general knowledge for recent events

    Test knowledge for remote events

Test for constructional ability

    Copy circle, cross, and cube; draw a clock

Test for ideomotor and ideational apraxia

    Perform tasks on command: complete complex sequence of actions

(continued)

6

TABLE 1–1.   **Bedside mental state testing** *(continued)*

Test executive function

   Verbal fluency: number of animals named in 1 minute or number of
     words that begin with a certain letter in 1 minute

   Perseveration: fist-palm-side test

Test for right-left disorientation

Test calculation

Test proverb interpretation

Test understanding of similarities

Retest memory: recall items of earlier memory tests

Test cognitive estimates

lance) are tested by reading to the patient a series of letters and asking him or her to tap every time a certain letter is called out.

Memory is tested clinically by immediate recall of digits, a sentence such as the Babcock sentence, four items given by the examiner, and items from a short story (standardized stories are available). Nonverbal learning can be tested by asking the patient to reproduce simple figures. Items of general knowledge should be tested, relevant to the patient's cultural and intellectual background. Tests of general knowledge about news items and about famous people or events should be given. The ability to accurately recall events from the more distant past (remote memory) should also be tested.

Testing for *aphasia* and *apraxia* is discussed in Chapter 5.

Anosognosia—denial of hemiparesis—most commonly accompanies right-hemisphere disease. *Finger agnosia* is the inability to recognize different fingers, either the patient's own or those of the examiner. *Autotopagnosia* is the same as finger agnosia, except that it applies to any body part. Finger agnosia and right-left disorientation usually indicate a left-hemisphere lesion.

Tests of constructional ability require the patient to draw a familiar object, such as a clock or a house. Poor performance, especially small or disorganized reproductions, suggest cerebral disease. *Neglect* of one-half of the drawing is seen with contralat-eral hemisphere lesions. Neglect is more common and more severe with right-hemisphere lesions.

Tests of *frontal lobe function* are often indicated in neuropsychi-atric patients. These are described in detail in Chapter 4, Table 4–1.

If possible, another person who knows the patient should be interviewed to confirm the accuracy of the patient's account of his or her illness. Family history should always be sought, and any potential genetic diseases should be noted. Anamnesis of early upbringing may reveal earlier behavior problems relevant to the clinical presentation. These include a history of sleepwalking, enuresis, stammering, tics, phobias, or hyperactivity. Developmen-tal delay, especially for motor development, speaking, and lan-guage, should be inquired about. *Attention-deficit disorder, conduct disorder, oppositional defiant disorder,* and *autistic behav-ior* should be noted.

NEUROLOGIC EXAMINATION

All patients should receive a neurologic examination. A screening examination for neurologic disease is shown in Table 1–2. This brief examination takes 10 minutes; if abnormalities are revealed, then more detailed testing is needed.

FORMAL TESTS OF NEUROPSYCHOLOGICAL FUNCTION

Formal tests of neuropsychological function are listed in Tables 1–3 and 4–1.

METABOLIC AND BIOCHEMICAL INVESTIGATIONS

The following tests are done for all patients:

- Hemoglobin, red blood cell count and related indices (hemato-crit, mean corpuscular volume [MCV], and mean corpuscular hemoglobin concentration [MCHC])

TABLE 1–2. **Brief neurologic screening examination**

Stance and gait

Observe walking and turning

Balance with feet together and eyes closed (Romberg's test)

Cranial nerves[a]

Smell (especially in head trauma) (I)

Check visual fields by quadrant (II)

Examine fundus (II)

Visual pursuit (III, IV, VI) (follow the examiner's finger in horizontal and vertical directions)

Bulk of temporalis and masseter muscles (V) (opening jaw against force; muscle bulk on tight bite)

Observe grimace of patient showing teeth (VII)

Rub finger and thumb an inch from the patient's ears for deafness (VIII)

Observe palate; ask patient to say "ah" (IX, X)

Push chin against the examiner's hand and test bulk of sternocleidomastoids (XI)

Observe tongue for abnormal movements or deviation on protrusion (XII)

Motor system

Test tone, power, and reflexes, and note muscle bulk (test in all four limbs)

Tone: hold arms out, palms down; observe any wrist drop; rotate leg at knee and note foot movements

Power: hold arms out, with palms down, and ask patient to "play the piano"; with palms up, watch for any flexion, pronation, or drift; elevate legs from couch and see whether they can be maintained in the air against examiner's pressure; tap floor rapidly with soles of the feet

Reflexes: muscle stretch (biceps, triceps, supinator, knee, ankle); pathological (plantar [Babinski sign])

Coordination

Finger-nose test

Rapid movements (tap quickly the back of one hand with the palm of the other)

(continued)

TABLE 1–2. **Brief neurologic screening examination**
            (continued)

Sensory testing

  Stroke skin on representative parts of the body, especially the distal
    extremities

Other reflexes

  Palmomental (draw a stick across the palm from the thenar eminence
    and watch for a reflex contraction of the ipsilateral mentalis muscle;
    the skin puckers)

  Grasp (stroke the patient's palm firmly moving outward)

  Jaw jerk

  Snout and pout reflexes (tap lips)

[a]Numeral in parentheses refers to the cranial nerve tested.

- White cell and platelet count
- Sedimentation rate
- Serum electrolytes (sodium and potassium chloride)
- Tests of liver function (alanine aminotransferase [ALT],
  alkaline phosphatase, aspartate aminotransferase [AST])
- Tests of renal function (blood urea nitrogen [BUN], urea)

The following tests are done for selected patients:

- Vitamin B_{12} and folic acid
- Iron and total iron-binding capacity
- Creatinine clearance test
- Calcium and phosphorus estimations
- Thyroid-stimulating hormone (TSH)
- Blood glucose; if abnormal, do extended glucose tolerance test
- Drug screen (for illicit drugs)
- Syphilis serology (Venereal Disease Research Laboratory
  [VDRL], fluorescent treponemal antibody absorption [FTA-ABS])
- Human immunodeficiency virus (HIV) serology, and T4 cell
  counts or T4-to-T8 ratio

TABLE 1–3. **Some formal neuropsychological tests**

Wechsler Adult Intelligence Scale (WAIS)—11 subtests, widely used to assess IQ

Halstead-Reitan Neuropsychological Test Battery—developed to detect structural lesions

Nelson Adult Reading Test (NART)—used to determine premorbid IQ

Wechsler Memory Scale—to test various components of memory

Progressive Matrices—a test of nonverbal intelligence, useful for those with language problems

Trail Making Test—patient connects ascending numbers (1, 2, etc.) and letters (a, b, etc.), then numbers alternating with letters (1-a, 2-b, etc.)

Wisconsin Card Sorting Test—tests patient's ability to infer rules and shift sets

---

- Prolactin—increased by neuroleptics; increased transiently by seizures
- Cholesterol and fatty acids
- Heavy metal screen

The following tests are done in association with specific diagnoses:

- Alcoholism: red cell transketolase, serum γ-glutamyltransferase (SGGT), serum alcohol
- Lupus (systemic lupus erythematosus [SLE]): lupus erythematosus cells and serum antinuclear or anti-DNA antibodies, antiphospholipid antibodies
- Fatigue: infectious mononucleosis (Paul Bunnel test), brucellosis (antibody titers)
- Polydipsia: plasma and urine osmolality
- Porphyria: urinary or fecal porphyrins
- Dexamethasone suppression test: see Table 1–4
- Dementia: see Chapter 9

- Movement disorders: serum copper and ceruloplasmin, serum creatine phosphokinase (CPK), acanthocytes in blood—see Chapter 10

The following tests are done for patients taking specific drugs:

- Lithium: routine lithium level
- Anticonvulsants: see Chapter 8, "Epilepsy and Limbic System Disorders"
- Antidepressants: levels are determined to check compliance or to detect unusual metabolism (e.g., patient complains of side effects on low doses)

Lumbar puncture is done to look for central nervous system (CNS) infections such as cerebral syphilis, to help in the differential diagnosis of dementia, and for the diagnosis of multiple sclerosis (oligoclonal bands).

THE ELECTROENCEPHALOGRAM

The electroencephalogram (EEG) was discovered by the psychiatrist Hans Berger. The EEG signal is created by the average of electrical currents from the surface dendrites of neurons.

The usual 10-20 system of electrode placement covers only 20% of the cortical surface. Additional electrodes, in the following placements, may improve the detection of abnormalities:

- Sphenoidal—in the region of the foramen ovale
- Nasopharyngeal—in the nasopharynx at the base of the skull
- Intracranial—subdural or intracerebral

Activation procedures facilitate detection of abnormal rhythms. These procedures include hyperventilation, photic stimulation, sleep induction or deprivation, and occasionally drugs (e.g., pentylenetetrazol).

TABLE 1–4. **Dexamethasone suppression test**

Day 1

Dexamethasone 1 mg orally at 11 P.M. (2300 h)

Day 2

Cortisol determinations at 8 A.M. (0800 h), 4 P.M. (1600 h), and 11 P.M. (2300 h)

Nonsuppression

Serum cortisol level of >5 μg/dl (138 nmol/L)

Causes of false-positive results

Medications

Benzodiazepines

Barbiturates

Hepatic enzyme-inducing anticonvulsants

Methadone, morphine

Indomethacin

Other drugs

Alcohol

Excess caffeine

Disease

Diabetes mellitus

Dementia

Cerebral tumor

Cardiac failure

Cushing's disease

Metabolic

Dehydration

Other

* Pregnancy

Acute trauma

Waveforms

There are four main types of waveforms:

- Alpha: 8–13 cycles per second (cps), maximal occipitally, blocked by eye opening

- Beta: faster than 13 cps, increased by many psychotropic drugs, especially sedatives and hypnotics
- Delta: below 4 cps, in the alert state often a sign of pathology
- Theta: 4–7 cps (Figure 1–1)

These waveforms are influenced by genetics, age, sleep, drugs, and disease. They do not correlate well with intelligence. Theta and delta waves are more common in the very young. Orthodox (non-rapid-eye-movement [NREM]) or slow-wave sleep is dominated by slow rhythms. Paradoxical (REM) sleep is characterized by fast desynchronized activity, similar to the waking recording, but the patient is asleep, and muscle activity is diminished.

During the night, there are usually six periods of REM sleep lasting up to 30 minutes, approximately 90 minutes apart—around 20%–25% of total sleep time. The first REM onset is after about

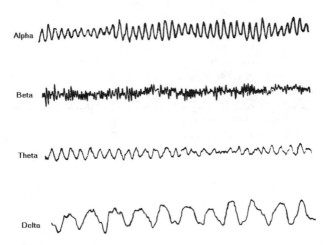

FIGURE 1–1. Typical electroencephalogram waveforms.
Source. Reprinted from Scott D: *Understanding EEG.* London, England, Duckworth, 1976, p. 24. Used with permission.

90 minutes (the REM latency). This period may be altered in disease states; for example, depressed patients have a short REM latency. Dreaming typically occurs during REM sleep.

The EEG is an important test in patients who present with paroxysmal behavioral disorders and in the workup of patients with epilepsy. Recordings during the period of the change or the ictus are of most value. The EEG is helpful in diagnosing tumors and some types of dementia and in delirium (see Chapter 9).

Evoked Potentials

The technique of evoked potentials allows the very small potentials generated by a stimulus to be exaggerated and studied. The results of many similar stimuli are averaged, and the signal-to-noise ratio is thus enhanced. The waveform is derived from computer analysis of the data; a series of positive and negative waves is detected. The latency (time from stimulus) of these waves is one index used to detect pathology. Usually, visual, auditory, or somatosensory evoked potentials are recorded.

Several potentials can be evoked by endogenous events. These include the contingent negative variation (CNV or expectancy wave), the P300 wave, and premotor potentials such as the Bereitschaft potential. The CNV arises out of anticipation of an expected response. It is a slow negative shift in the vertex and frontal regions. The P300 wave is thought to relate to a process of cognitive appraisal of a stimulus.

Other EEG Techniques

Ambulatory monitoring involves placing electrodes on the head (or heart), signals from which are continuously recorded onto a small cassette recorder that patients attach to themselves. Patients can walk around wearing this recorder, and recordings over days can be made, for example, in the home. With *videotelemetry,* a picture of patients' behavior is recorded simultaneously with their EEG, and both are replayed side by side on a television screen. The behavior and the EEG can be directly compared.

Computerized EEG mapping produces topographical images of the brain's electrical activity by means of computerized analysis of the various EEG components.

Magnetoencephalography

Magnetoencephalography, which detects magnetic source fields in the brain, complements EEG. However, because magnetic signals are not interfered with by the skull, magnetoencephalography provides better spatial resolution and detects fields beneath the surface.

BRAIN IMAGING

Skull X Rays

Skull X rays are of little value when other imaging techniques are available.

Computed Tomography

Computed tomography (CT) provides a computerized image of brain structure. It is essential to obtain a structural image of the brain in any patient suspected of having a focal cerebral lesion. CT also helps in the evaluation of many other conditions—for example, dementia, in which more diffuse pathology is expected.

In CT, X rays are projected through the brain in many directions around the patient's head. Those X rays interacting with intrinsic brain electrons are captured or scattered and do not reach the detectors, the number detected depending on the tissue density. This allows a matrix display of brain density, represented as squares that reflect the average density of the tissue lying within the imaged area. The square is the pixel; the volume of tissue represented is the voxel.

The *partial volume effect* is an important source of error. If a voxel contains an admixture of tissue and air or tissue and bone, the average result may suggest pathology where none is present.

Contrast media are given that are efficient at electron capture, delete X rays, and enhance the image of pathological tissue.

CT remains the first examination of choice in many centers, especially where magnetic resonance imaging (MRI) is unavailable. It should always be requested if there is any suspicion of intracranial pathology.

Magnetic Resonance Imaging

The principle of MRI is examination of the physicochemical environment of the brain's protons.

An object (proton) with a charge and velocity provokes a magnetic field adjacent to it. Because protons spin around their axis at random, the sum total of magnetization in an area of the brain is zero. On application of an external magnetic field, the particles and their charges align, just like the compass needle of a small compass in the earth's magnetic field.

The aligned protons can now be excited by the momentary application of a radio signal at their specific frequency, a process likened to a tuning fork provoking resonation in a guitar string tuned to it. When the signal is turned off, a signal is returned (i.e., the guitar string continues to resonate), which can be detected and analyzed. Thus, after the application of the radiofrequency pulse, the magnetization returns exponentially to its preexcitement level: the relaxation. This process is defined by two time constants known as T1 and T2. A T1-weighted image is referred to as the inversion recovery image. The T2 image is referred to as the spin-spin relaxation time. A variant image is the spin echo.

Each tissue has specific T1 and T2 values. In the brain, the measured proton behavior relates to the hydrogen nucleus, most commonly water. By exploiting relaxation times of different tissues, heightened contrast between these tissues is achieved.

The derived image has a low spatial resolution (in some machines, <1.0 mm^2).

Most pathologic tissues increase the length of T1 and T2. On T1 images, this lengthening is darker; on T2 images, it is lighter.

The advantages and disadvantages of MRI are shown in Table 1–5.

Magnetic resonance spectroscopy (MRS) refers to a quantitation of the physicochemical spectra that are derived from MRI. The main techniques are phosphorus-31 MRS, which gives information about membrane phospholipid and high-energy phosphate metabolism; and H1 (proton) MRS, with a broader spectrum encompassing choline and some amino acids, including some neurotransmitters such as glutamate and γ-aminobutyric acid (GABA). Different disease states produce different chemical changes in the brain that may be detected by MRS.

More modern techniques allow good quantitation of neuronal structures; for example, they allow accurate assessment of hippocampal volumes. It is also possible to capture functional images *(functional or echoplanar MRI)*. This technique relies on the principle that active neurons convert more hemoglobin to oxyhemoglobin, increasing the relaxation time (T2); determination of this ratio over two closely related periods provides an assessment of blood flow.

Single Photon Emission Computed Tomography and Positron Emission Tomography

In contrast to the above imaging methods (which, apart from newer MRI techniques, assess brain structure), single photon emission computed tomography (SPECT) and positron-emission tomography (PET) assess brain function.

Cerebral blood flow (CBF) and *metabolism* are normally closely linked; hence, assessment of CBF may provide an indirect measure of neuronal activity. In SPECT, a patient is given a dose of a radioactive tracer that specifically interacts with brain tissue. Commonly used is technetium-99m HMPAO, which is taken up by tissue and then trapped. Radiation is detected by rotating gamma cameras, and, by a process of backprojection and tomographic reconstruction, an image of blood flow is obtained. SPECT and PET are contrasted in Table 1–6.

TABLE 1–5. **Advantages and disadvantages of magnetic resonance imaging**

Advantages	Disadvantages
No radiation	Noise discomfort
Minimal risk[a]	Claustrophobia
Good gray/white contrast	Limited discrimination between pathologies
Less degradation of image with movement	Length of scan time
No bone artifacts	Artifacts from ferromagnetic material (e.g., tooth fillings)
Clear structural images	Expensive
Ability to visualize several planes	Limited availability
Very sensitive to some types of pathology	

[a]Patients with cardiac pacemakers or intracranial magnetic clips or in the first trimester of pregnancy should not be scanned.

PET is primarily a research instrument. Radioactive isotopes are created by a cyclotron. These essentially are compounds that gain a proton, which becomes unstable. In tissue, the proton unites with an electron, and the two particles convert their mass into radiation energy. They annihilate, releasing two coincident gamma rays at 180 degrees to each other. These are detected by a scanner,

TABLE 1–6. **Comparison of PET and SPECT**

Characteristic	PET	SPECT
Cost	Expensive	Less expensive
Resolution (mm)	3–5	6–10
Availability	Very limited	Limited
Acquisition time	Seconds	Minutes
Cyclotron source	On site	Need not be on site
Isotope range	More versatile	Less versatile

Note. PET = positron-emission tomography. SPECT = single photon emission computed tomography.

and, via computerized reconstruction of the data, an image is created.

Several different positron emitters are available, but most work is done with carbon-11, fluorine-18, and oxygen-15. The resulting images are of CBF or metabolism.

With both PET and SPECT, it is possible to label ligands for a variety of drugs and neuroreceptors, for example, the D_2 receptor.

■ REFERENCES AND RECOMMENDED READING

Andreasen NC (section ed): Brain imaging, in American Psychiatric Press Review of Psychiatry, Vol 12. Edited by Oldham JM, Riba MB, Tasman A. Washington, DC, American Psychiatric Press, 1993, pp 315–510

George MS, Ring HA, Costa DC, et al: Neuroactivation and Neuroimaging with SPECT. New York, Springer-Verlag, 1991

Grant I, Adams KM: Neuropsychological Assessment of Neuropsychiatric Disorders, 2nd Edition. New York, Oxford University Press, 1994

Roberts JKA: Differential Diagnosis in Neuropsychiatry. Chichester, UK, Wiley, 1984

Rosse RB, Giese AA, Deutch SI, et al: Concise Guide to Laboratory and Diagnostic Testing in Psychiatry. Washington, DC, American Psychiatric Press, 1989

Strub RL, Black FW: The Mental Status Examination in Neurology, 3rd Edition. Philadelphia, PA, FA Davis, 1993

Trimble MR: Biological Psychiatry, 2nd Edition. Chichester, UK, Wiley, 1994

BEHAVIORAL NEUROBIOLOGY

2

■ NEUROPHYSIOLOGY AND NEUROCHEMISTRY

To understand the somatic underpinnings of neuropsychiatric illness, it necessary to know basic neuroanatomic and neurochemical principles.

The brain is composed of *neurons* and *glial cells.* The main link between neurons is the synapse. The *synaptic cleft* is around 20 nm wide, and *neurotransmitters* are released from the *presynaptic* to the *postsynaptic* membrane. Calcium is essential for neurotransmitter release.

There are four main ions in cells: sodium, potassium, chloride, and organic anions. The *resting potential* is maintained by the action of the sodium pump that forces sodium out and draws potassium into the cell. This is the energy store of the cell. The *action potential* is generated by the influx of sodium and the loss of potassium during synaptic transmission, and the resulting current is propagated along the cell membrane.

Postsynaptic potentials are either inhibitory (IPPS) or excitatory (EPPS), and these summate to determine the ultimate excitability of the postsynaptic cell.

Receptors are proteins to which neurotransmitters and other *ligands* bind. Many receptors in the central nervous system (CNS) have been cloned, and their structures have been identified. Once a transmitter has interacted with a receptor, either ion exchange occurs with alteration of the membrane potential or there is stimulation of a *secondary messenger,* which may then alter intracellular metabolism. Adenylate cyclase, generating cyclic adenosine monophosphate (cAMP), is one common system. Genes such as c-*fos* may be switched on.

22

Many receptors have been described, but the main ones of relevance are shown in Table 2–1.

Neurons have a soma, an axon, dendrites, and synapses. Tubulin, a protein in the axon, acts in the transport of molecules down the axon. Larger axons are surrounded by a myelin sheath that increases the speed of conduction.

TABLE 2–1. **Neuroreceptors of clinical relevance**

Receptor	Subtypes	Comments
Dopamine	5	D_2 is related to movement disorder; all neuroleptics bind to it; antipsychotic effect of typical neuroleptics is related to intensity of binding; abundant in striatum D_1 has possible relevance in psychosis D_4: clozapine has good affinity
Norepinephrine	α, β	Predominant in cortex, limbic system, and striatum α_2 linked to depression
Serotonin (5-HT)	4	5-HT_{1a} linked to anxiety 5-HT_{1d} linked to migraine 5-HT_2 linked to depression 5-HT_3 linked to memory
GABA	A, B	Linked to the benzodiazepine receptor; on activation, chloride channels open; inhibitory; abundant all over brain; type A linked to seizures and anxiety
Acetylcholine	Nicotinic, muscarinic	Linked to memory and cognition
Peptide	Many	Includes opiate-binding sites
Glutamate	NMDA, AMPA	Related to seizures

Note. Many of these receptors have subtypes not noted here.
AMPA = α-amino-3-hydroxy-5-methyl-4-isoxazole propionic acid.
GABA = γ-aminobutyric acid. NMDA = *N*-methyl-D-aspartate.

There are five types of glial cells: astrocytes, oligodendrocytes, microglia, Schwann cells, and ependymal cells. These cells provide structural phagocytic and metabolic support for neurons and manufacture myelin.

The main *neurotransmitters* are shown in Table 2–2. Many others are known to exist, but their function is poorly understood. These include peptides such as the enkephalins, substance P, and cholecystokinin. In individual neurons, two or more neurotransmitters may coexist.

Dopamine is related to the control of movement and to psychosis, γ-aminobutyric acid (GABA) to seizure activity, *serotonin* to impulse control and mood, and *acetylcholine* to memory.

TABLE 2–2. **Some neurotransmitters**

Neurotransmitter	Synthesized from	Metabolite	Main location
Acetylcholine	Choline	Acetyl-CoA	Spinal cord Caudate Hippocampus Nucleus of Meynert
Dopamine	Tyrosine	Homovanillic acid	Substantia nigra Ventral tegmental area Basal ganglia Limbic system
GABA and glutamate	Glutamate	Glutamic acid	Ubiquitous Cortical/subcortical
Norepinephrine	Tyrosine	MHPG	Locus coeruleus Limbic system Cortex
Serotonin (5-HT)	Tryptophan	5-HIAA	Raphe nucleus Limbic system Cortex

Note. GABA = γ-aminobutyric acid. 5-HIAA = 5-hydroxyindoleacetic acid. MHPG = 3-methoxy-4-hydroxyphenylglycol.

■ ESSENTIAL NEUROANATOMY

LIMBIC SYSTEM

The limbic system is involved in the experience of emotion, and its integrity is essential for emotional well-being. Alteration of the structure or function of the limbic system is found in many neuropsychiatric illnesses.

The main nuclei and pathways of the limbic system are shown in Table 2–3. The cortex of the limbic system proper (archicortex, allocortex) is three layered, as opposed to the six layers of the neocortex (Table 2–4). Intermediate is the mesocortex.

Common characteristics of limbic structures are connection to the hypothalamus and association with the amygdala and hippocampus. The connections from the midbrain nuclei, which are the origin of neurotransmitters so relevant to the regulation of behavior, to the forebrain structures such as the nucleus accumbens are referred to as the *mesolimbic system.* The orbitofrontal cortex is also included as part of the limbic circuitry.

Figure 2–1 outlines the most important structures of the limbic system. The *amygdala* is related to the control of aggression, to

TABLE 2–3. **Limbic system**

Main nuclei	Main gyri	Main pathway
Amygdala	Cingulate	Fornix
Septal	Parahippocampal	Stria terminalis
Hypothalamic	Hippocampal	Cingulum
Anterior and medio-	Dentate	Mammilothalamic tract
dorsal thalamic		Medial forebrain bundle
Mamillary bodies		
Nucleus accumbens		
Raphe		
Ventral tegmental area		
Locus coeruleus		

TABLE 2–4. **Layers of the cerebral cortex**

Layer	Layer name	Structure
I	Molecular	Contains the terminal dendritic ramifications of cells from deeper layers
II	External granular	Small, closely packed neurons with dendrites in layer I and axons in the deeper layers
III	External pyramidal	Pyramidal neurons with apical dendrites in layer I and axons that comprise association and commissural fibers of white matter
IV	Internal granular	Densely packed stellate neurons with axons that ramify within the layer or descend to deeper layers and white matter; this layer receives projections from the sensory thalamic nuclei and forms the cortex's "window" on the external world
V	Internal pyramidal	Large and medium-sized pyramidal neurons whose dendrites arborize in layers I, IV, and V; axons form projection fibers
VI	Fusiform	Spindle-shaped neurons with dendrites in layers I, IV, and VI; axons are projection fibers or short association (U connecting adjacent sulci) fibers

affective tone of incoming sensations, to anxiety, to learning associations between stimuli and reinforcement, and possibly to psychosis.

The *hippocampus* plays a major role in memory.

The *parahippocampal gyrus* (a part of which is referred to as the *entorhinal cortex*) is a meeting point where sensory information from the outside world integrates with data from the inside of the organism. Thus, sensory information first reaches the cortex at *unimodal primary sensory areas*. It is then projected to *secondary*

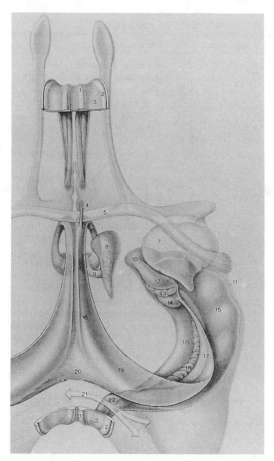

FIGURE 2–1. Limbic system structures from above, isolated from their surroundings. 5 = anterior commisure; 7 = amygdala; 8 = anterior nucleus of the thalamus; 9 = mammillothalamic tract; 10 = subiculum; 12 = Ammons horn; 15 = hippocampus; 16 = fornix; and 19 = fornix. *Source.* For complete text and remaining key, see Nieuwenhuys R, Voogd J, van Huijzen Chr: *The Human Nervous System*, 3rd Edition. Heidelberg, Germany, Springer-Verlag, 1988, p. 300. Reprinted with permission. Copyright 1988 Springer-Verlag.

sensory areas, and then to *multimodal association cortex.* These
cortical regions project to the parahippocampal gyrus (Figure 2–2),
providing integrated sensory information. This information is further projected to hippocampal structures and the amygdala. The
latter two in turn influence and are influenced by information on
the internal state of the organism derived from hypothalamic and
other subcortical limbic structures. The hypothalamus has extensive connections with the visceral nuclei in the brain stem.

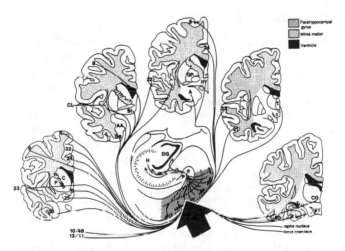

FIGURE 2–2. Projections to the parahippocampal gyrus. Those shown are from
the same hemisphere, but smaller projections also exist from the opposite hemisphere. A = amygdala; C = caudate; CG = central gray; DG = gyrus dentate; GP =
globus pallidus; H = hippocampus; HY = hypothalamus; I = insula; P = putamen;
PP = perforant path; S = septum; SI = substantia innominata; T = thalamus; and
VT = ventral tegmentum. For complete text and remaining key, see Roberts GW,
Horton K: "Neuropathology of Psychoses," in *The Temporal Lobes and the Limbic
System.* Edited by Trimble MR, Bolwig TG. Petersfield, England, Wrightson Biomedical, p. 221. *Source.* Reprinted from Roberts GW: "Schizophrenia: A Neuropathological Perspective." *British Journal of Psychiatry* 158:8–17, 1991. Used
with permission.

The *cingulate gyrus* is an extensive cortical gyrus that is part of the so-called *Papez circuit.* The Papez circuit consists of *hippocampus—mamillary bodies—anterior thalamic nucleus—cingulate gyrus—hippocampus.* The circuit is the core structure of the limbic system.

The cingulate gyrus is involved in some highly complex mammalian activities, such as maternal behavior, play, pain, and attention. It is sometimes lesioned in neurosurgical procedures to treat obsessive-compulsive disorder (OCD), pain, and depression.

BASAL GANGLIA

The *basal ganglia* typically include the *caudate nucleus, putamen,* and *globus pallidus.* The *striatum* refers to the caudate and the putamen, the former being a large C-shaped nucleus that adheres throughout its length to the lateral ventricles and is continuous anteriorly with the putamen.

Medially, within the head of the caudate nucleus is the *nucleus accumbens.* The nucleus accumbens and some adjacent dopamine-rich nuclei are sometimes referred to as the *ventral* or *limbic striatum.*

It is now appreciated that the basal ganglia are members of brain circuits that mediate cognitive as well as motor processes. Five frontal-subcortical circuits have been described that link specific frontal regions with the basal ganglia and thalamus. The five loops originate in the supplementary motor cortex, the frontal eye fields, the dorsolateral prefrontal cortex, the orbitofrontal cortex, and the anterior cingulate cortex, respectively. The three behaviorally relevant circuits are shown in Figure 2–3. Each circuit has sequential connections between the frontal lobes, caudate or putamen, globus pallidus and substantia nigra, and thalamus, as well as an indirect pathway (not shown) that interposes connections between the subthalamic nucleus and the globus pallidus externa and the globus pallidus interna before rejoining the direct pathway. Thus, the main outflow from the caudate and putamen occurs via

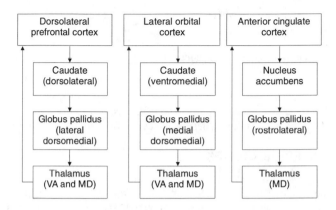

FIGURE 2–3. Frontal-subcortical circuits. The three circuits relevant to behavior are shown. Injury to the dorsolateral prefrontal circuit produces executive dysfunction, damage to the orbitofrontal circuit causes disinhibition, and dysfunction of the medial frontal circuit produces apathy. VA = ventral anterior nucleus; MD = medial dorsal nucleus. *Source.* Reprinted from Cummings JL: "Frontal-Subcortical Circuits and Human Behavior." *Archives of Neurology* 50:873–880, 1993 (Figure 2, p. 875). Copyright 1993 American Medical Association. Used with permission.

the globus pallidus, which then connects to the thalamus. The ventral striatum flows to the *ventral pallidum,* and then also to the *thalamus.* The ventral pallidum is sometimes called the *substantia innominata,* an area rich in acetylcholine and associated with the *basal nucleus of Meynert.*

The most important loops for emotional behavior involve the ventral striatum, which has limbic connections. The substantia nigra-caudate pathway is involved in Parkinson's disease. These frontal-subcortical circuits provide an explanation for the similarities between the behavioral abnormalities that accompany frontal lobe dysfunction and those that occur with basal ganglia and thalamic injury.

Of great importance for neuropsychiatry is the influence of the limbic system on the basal ganglia. The ventral striatum is one of the crossroads where emotional and motoric information can influence each other.

RETICULAR ACTIVATING SYSTEM

The *reticular activating system* (RAS) is a large collection of fibers and nuclei that include the main monoamine nuclei, extending from the medulla oblongata to the thalamus. Structures within the RAS modulate arousal, sleep-wake cycles, and conscious activity.

CEREBRAL CORTEX

The *cerebral cortex* is traditionally numbered after the scheme devised by Brodmann. The four lobes—frontal, parietal, occipital, and temporal—are defined solely on the basis of surface markings (see Figure 2–4). The cortex has a large number of association fibers that link areas of the same hemisphere and commissural fibers that link homotopic areas of the two hemispheres. The largest of these is the *corpus callosum.*

The primary somatosensory cortex is located posterior to the central sulcus in the postcentral gyrus. More posteriorly is the somatic sensory association area. The auditory cortical areas are in the superior temporal gyrus, and the visual areas are in the striate cortex.

The main motor cortex is in the precentral gyrus, immediately rostral to the central sulcus.

The *frontal lobes* are represented anatomically by those areas anterior to the central sulcus. The motor strip is Brodmann area 4; the premotor area is in front of the motor strip (areas 6, 44, and 45). The frontal eye field is Brodmann area 8. The supplementary motor area is Brodmann area 6, on the medial aspect of the hemisphere.

The *prefrontal cortex* designates the anterior portion of the frontal lobe. It is divided into the dorsolateral prefrontal cortex (Brodmann areas 9, 10, and 46), the medial frontal cortex (Brodmann area 24; anterior cingulate cortex), and the orbitofrontal cortex (Brodmann areas 11 and 12).

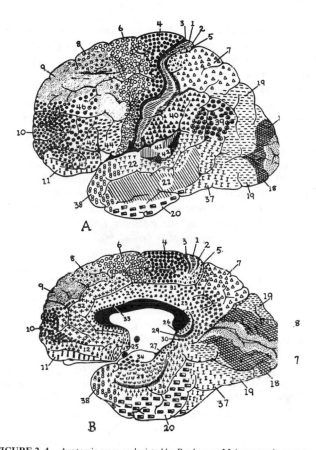

FIGURE 2–4. Anatomic areas as depicted by Brodmann. Main anatomic areas to note are the following: 1, 2, and 3 = primary somatosensory areas; 4 = primary motor cortex; 6 = premotor area; 8, 9, 10, 11, 12, 45, 46, and 47 = prefrontal granular cortex; 17 = visual cortex; 22 = superior temporal gyrus; 23, 24, 31, and 33 = cingulate gyrus; 27, 28, and 34 = parahippocampal gyrus; 38 = temporal pole; 39 and 40 = inferior parietal lobule; and 41 and 42 = auditory cortex (Heschle's gyri). *Source.* Reprinted from Carpenter MB: *Core Text of Neuroanatomy,* 4th Edition. Baltimore, MD, Williams & Wilkins, 1991, p. 399. Used with permission.

The frontal lobes are six-layered neocortex, and the motor and premotor areas are agranular cortex. Layers III and V contain the long projection fibers that descend from these areas to the brain stem and spinal cord and are enlarged compared with other cortical regions. The prefrontal cortex is granular cortex: layers II and IV are larger and layers III and V are smaller than the cortex of the motor and premotor areas. The caudal orbitofrontal cortex and the cingulate cortex of the frontal lobes are paralimbic regions, composed of mesocortex, transitional between the archicortex (three layered) and the neocortex (six layered).

The frontal lobes receive afferent association fibers from other cortical areas and projections from subcortical structures. In addition, each frontal lobe receives commissural fibers from the contralateral frontal areas. The prefrontal cortex receives fibers from unimodal association cortex (visual, auditory, somatesthetic) and posterior heteromodal cortex of the inferior parietal lobule. These projections are reciprocal and are distributed in the *superior longitudinal fasciculus.* Fibers from the amygdala and medial temporal cortex enter the prefrontal regions via the *uncinate fasciculus.* The principal subcortical projections to the prefrontal cortex originate in the *medial dorsal nucleus of the thalamus.* Afferent connections from the hypothalamus are also present. Thus, the prefrontal cortex receives sensory information from the posterior cortical regions and limbic input from temporal, thalamic, and hypothalamic structures, creating the opportunity for the integration of environmental, emotional, and interoceptive information.

The efferent connections of the frontal lobes include reciprocal connections with the sources of afferent input from other cortical and subcortical regions. These connections create the opportunity for the frontal lobes to modulate and modify their own input. In addition, the frontal cortex has unidirectional projections to the head of the caudate nucleus, nucleus accumbens, and putamen. Connections to the hypothalamus are largely efferent in nature. The final output of the nervous system is mediated by frontobulbar connections and frontospinal connections descending to brain stem and spinal cord nuclei in the pyramidal tract. It is via this tract that humans effect environmental change, through speech and movement.

The frontal-subcortical projections use glutamate as their principal transmitter. However, the afferents to the frontal cortex include extensive dopamine, noradrenergic, and serotonergic neurons from the midbrain and pons. The nucleus basalis also provides cholinergic input. GABA, an inhibitory transmitter, is present in high concentrations in the cerebral cortex.

THE CEREBELLUM

The *cerebellum* lies posteriorly over the brain stem. Its cortex is divided into the central vermis and the cerebellar hemispheres. Recently, direct links between this structure and the limbic system have been found.

Some important associations between neuroanatomic sites and behavior are listed in Table 2–5.

TABLE 2–5.   **Some brain-behavior associations**

Structure	Behavior
Cingulate gyrus	Maternal behavior, play, vocalization, attention, pain, motivation
Hippocampus	Memory, anxiety
Amygdala	Fear, anxiety, aggression, sexual behavior, psychosis, mood
Septum	Pleasure, addiction
Hypothalamus	Eating, drinking, sex, aggression, hormonal regulation
Reticular activating system	Arousal, sleep-wake cycle
Entorhinal cortex	Memory, sensory integration
Ventral striatum	Motivation

■ BRAIN-BEHAVIOR RELATIONSHIPS

Theories of *localization* implied that specific mental functions resided in specific locations in the brain. *Lateralization* implies that some functions are predominantly mediated by one hemisphere or the other. *Theories of equipotentiality* denied such localization, whereas the concept of *parallel distributed processing* (PDP) seeks an intermediate ground. PDP implies the existence of integrated neuronal circuits that are widely distributed in the brain and have the capacity to change their response bias with learning. Any point in the circuit may interconnect with other circuits; hence, there can be multiple potential effects from a single lesion. Likewise, similar effects could emerge from lesions in different parts of the same circuit.

■ REFERENCES AND RECOMMENDED READING

Aggleton JP (ed): The Amygdala. New York, Wiley-Liss, 1992

Alexander GE, DeLong MR, Strick PL: Parallel organisation of functionally segregated circuits linking basal ganglia and cortex. Annu Rev Neurosci 9:357–381, 1986

Cummings JL: Fronto-subcortical circuits and human behavior. Arch Neurol 50:873–880, 1993

Fuster JM: The Prefrontal Cortex, 2nd Edition. New York, Raven, 1989

Heimer L, Switzer RD, VanHoesen GW: Ventral striatum and ventral pallidum. Trends in Neuroscience 5:83–87, 1982

MacLean PD: The Triune Brain in Evolution. New York, Plenum, 1990

Mesulam M-M: Patterns in behavioral anatomy: association areas, the limbic system, and hemispheric specialization, in Principles of Behavioral Neurology. Edited by Mesulam M-M. Philadelphia, PA, FA Davis, 1985, pp 1–70

Nauta WHT, Domesick VB: Neural associations of the limbic system, in The Neural Basis of Behavior. Edited by Beckman A. New York, Spectrum, 1982, pp 175–206

Stuss DT, Benson DF: The Frontal Lobes. New York, Raven, 1986

Weinberger DR: A connectionist approach to the prefrontal cortex. J Neuropsychiatry Clin Neurosci 5:241–253, 1993

NEUROPSYCHIATRIC SYMPTOMS AND SYNDROMES

Neuropsychiatric diagnosis is based on elicitation of clinical symptoms, identification of neuropsychiatric syndromes, construction of a differential diagnosis, use of laboratory tests and neuroimaging to support or exclude specific diagnoses, and identification of the primary etiology of the behavioral disturbance. In some cases, longitudinal assessment and careful monitoring of treatment responses may be necessary to clarify obscure diagnoses. Treatment depends on accurate diagnosis.

This chapter addresses neuropsychiatric symptoms and syndromes and the differential diagnosis of the major neuropsychiatric disorders. Available information on the pathophysiology of each syndrome is reviewed. The syndromes described include depression, mania, mood and affect lability, delusions, hallucinations, anxiety, obsessive-compulsive disorder and other repetitive behaviors, personality changes indicative of brain dysfunction, dissociative disorders, and altered sexual behavior. Definitions of these syndromes are provided in Chapter 1. Neuropsychiatric syndromes associated with frontal lobe disorders are described in more detail in Chapter 4, and symptoms and syndromes indicative of epilepsy and limbic system dysfunction are described more extensively in Chapter 8. Treatment of neuropsychiatric disorders is discussed in the relevant disease-oriented chapters (Chapters 8–13) and is summarized in Chapter 14.

■ DEPRESSION

Depression has mood, affective, cognitive, behavioral, neurovegetative, and endocrine dimensions. *Mood* changes in depression include sadness and loss of the ability to experience pleasure. Anxiety is common in depression. *Affect* refers to the outward expression of internal mood states and in depression is characterized by a restricted range of emotional display, weeping and tearfulness, and a sad or concerned demeanor. *Cognitive alterations* characteristic of depression include loss of motivation with apathy and diminished initiative. In addition, the patients express thoughts of worthlessness, hopelessness, and helplessness. They may be preoccupied with thoughts of guilt or concerns about personal health (i.e., hypochondriasis). Many patients note decreased ability to concentrate, and some develop a dementia syndrome (e.g., dementia syndrome of depression). Withdrawal and disinterest in social interactions are common. Some patients evidence mood-congruent hallucinations (e.g., believe that they smell rotting substances) and delusions (e.g., believe that they have cancer or are guilty of serious offenses). *Behavioral ramifications* of depression feature changes in vocal expression and body movement. Patients are often hypophonic and have a diminished range of vocal intensity. They may have psychomotor retardation or agitation. *Neurovegetative changes* in depression include altered sleep patterns (early morning awakening, multiple nocturnal awakenings, difficulty falling asleep, hypersomnia, decreased rapid eye movement [REM] latency), appetite alterations (decreased or increased), excessive fatigue, and diminished libido. *Endocrine abnormalities* that occur in some depressed patients encompass changes in the hypothalamic-pituitary-adrenal axis and the hypothalamic-pituitary-thyroid axis. There may be excessive cortisol secretion and a failure to suppress serum cortisol in response to orally administered dexamethasone in the dexamethasone suppression test (DST; see Table 1–4); in addition, there may a blunted response to thyrotropin-releasing hormone (TRH) manifested by an abnormally small rise in thyroid-stimulating hormone (TSH).

Patients with major depressive episodes have changes in most of the above-listed domains during the same 2-week period. Patients with dysthymic disorder have less severe changes that persist for longer periods (at least 2 years or essentially continuously since the onset of a brain disorder).

Depression has been linked to a wide variety of brain diseases and is the most common major neuropsychiatric complication of brain dysfunction (Table 3–1). The treatable nature of depression makes it imperative that depression be sought and actively treated in patients with brain disorders.

Review of the disorders in Table 3–1 reveals that depression is linked to dysfunction in specific brain regions. Disorders affecting the frontal lobes, temporal lobes, and basal ganglia (especially the caudate nuclei) are particularly likely to be accompanied by depressive syndromes. Involvement of the left frontal lobe or left caudate nucleus is more likely than right-sided dysfunction to precipitate depression, and depression is more severe and more frequent the closer the left frontal lesion is to the frontal pole. Serotonergic, noradrenergic, and dopaminergic transmitter systems are implicated in the pathogenesis of depression; and abnormalities of motivation, stress response, and behavioral programming mediated by frontal-subcortical circuits are involved in many of the symptoms of the depression syndrome.

Depression is treated with monocyclic or heterocyclic antidepressants, selective serotonin reuptake inhibitors, monoamine oxidase inhibitors, or electroconvulsive therapy (Chapter 14).

■ MANIA

The manic syndrome is comprised of abnormalities of mood, affect, cognition, motor activity, and neurovegetative function. *Mood changes* typical of the manic patient include euphoria, lability, and irritability. Depressive symptoms are commonly mixed with the expansive, elevated mood state to create a mixed mood abnormality. *Affective alterations* are characterized by excessive laughter, smiling, and marked animation. *Cognitive changes* include racing thoughts, flight of ideas, grandiosity, poor judgment with risk taking, and unrestrained enthusiasm for poorly conceived business or social schemes. Cognitive disorganization and distractibility with impaired ability to concentrate are frequently present.

TABLE 3–1. **Depression occurring in conjunction with neurologic disorders**

Neurologic condition	Frequency of depressive syndromes (%)[a]	Characteristics of the depressive syndrome
Stroke	30–60	Psychomotor retardation often severe; depression more common in patients with brain atrophy; depression most frequent with left frontal and left caudate lesions; symptoms most severe as lesion approaches the left frontal pole
Parkinson's disease	30–50	Anxiety is commonly present; delusions and suicide are rare; PET reveals diminished orbitofrontal and caudate glucose metabolism
Huntington's disease	35–45	Suicide is common; PET reveals diminished orbitofrontal glucose metabolism
Epilepsy	10–50	Frequency of suicide and delusions is increased; PET reveals diminished orbitofrontal glucose metabolism
Traumatic brain injury	25–50	A history of psychiatric disorder (including substance abuse) is more common among the patients who develop posttraumatic depression
Multiple sclerosis	25–50	Depression is not related to the degree of disability
Alzheimer's disease	30–40	Major depressive episodes are rare
Vascular dementia	25–60	Depression is common in lacunar state and Binswanger's disease

Note. PET = positron-emission tomography.
[a]Depressive disorders include both major depressive episodes and less severe symptomatic depression syndromes.

Estimations of self-worth are inflated. Mood-congruent delusions (e.g., delusions of having special powers or abilities) and hallucinations may be present. *Motoric manifestations* of mania include hyperactivity, hypersexuality, and excessive talkativeness. Speech may be loud and excessively fast. The patient is often intrusive, domineering, and discourteous in social interactions. *Neurovegetative dysfunction* in mania features insomnia, increased appetite, increased libido, and enhanced energy. Hypomania has many of the same features as mania, but the symptoms are less severe and do not cause impaired social or occupational function.

Mania and hypomania have been associated with a variety of neurologic conditions (Table 3–2). Nearly all the focal lesions that produce mania are located in the right hemisphere and involve the orbitofrontal cortex, caudate nuclei, thalamus or perithalamic regions, or the basotemporal area. Mood modulation, hypothalamic control of neurovegetative functions, and limbic system activities are disrupted in manic syndromes.

Mania and hypomania are treated with lithium, carbamazepine, clonazepam, or valproic acid (Chapter 14).

TABLE 3 2. **Neurologic disorders associated with mania or hypomania**

Stroke (most common with right-brain lesions and in patients with a family history of psychiatric illness)

Parkinson's disease after dopaminergic therapy

Huntington's disease

Idiopathic basal ganglia calcification (Fahr's disease)

Traumatic brain injury

Multiple sclerosis

Epilepsy (peri-ictal)

Frontotemporal dementias

General paresis (syphilitic encephalitis)

■ MOOD AND AFFECT LABILITY

Lability of mood refers to the rapid shift of one mood state to another. This shift is typical of patients with lesions of the orbitofrontal cortex such as traumatic brain injury, orbitofrontal meningiomas, frontal degenerations, and encephalopathies after rupture of anterior communicating artery aneurysms. Lability is also present in some basal ganglia disorders including Huntington's disease and idiopathic basal ganglia calcification (Fahr's disease).

Lability of affect refers to sudden changes in emotional expression. The affect may be mood incongruent or may be greatly in excess of the associated mood changes. Pseudobulbar palsy, affective abnormalities occurring in the course of epileptic seizures, and affect dysregulation in Angelman's syndrome produce affective lability. The *pseudobulbar palsy* syndrome includes excessive laughter or weeping without concomitant mood changes, dysarthria, dysphagia, facial paresis, increased gag reflex, and increased jaw jerk. Brisk limb reflexes, spasticity, and Babinski signs are frequently evident on neurologic examination. The pseudobulbar palsy syndrome reflects disruption of descending corticobulbar tracts above the level of the mid-pons and occurs with stroke (particularly lacunar state and Binswanger's disease), multiple sclerosis, amyotrophic lateral sclerosis, trauma, and tumors of the base of the skull. Pseudobulbar affect has been successfully treated with amitriptyline, amantadine, levodopa, and fluoxetine.

Epileptic seizures may be manifested by alterations in affect. *Gelastic epilepsy* refers to seizures featuring laughter as an ictal automatism; *dacrystic epilepsy* comprises ictal crying or tearing. Ictal changes in affect are typically accompanied by other seizure manifestations including altered consciousness, limb movements, and electroencephalographic (EEG) changes. Ictal affect abnormalities occur most commonly as manifestations of partial complex seizures in patients with temporal lobe epilepsy. *Infantile spasms* may also be accompanied by prolonged laughter or short attacks of giggling or grinning. Finally, ictal laughter may occur with lesions of the hypothalamus. Precocious puberty, chiasmal blindness, and central fever may accompany hypothalamic seizures. Ictal affective changes respond to treatment with anticon vulsants.

Angelman's syndrome is characterized by developmental delay, absent speech, ataxia with puppetlike jerky movements, paroxysms of unprovoked laughter, and dysmorphic features (microcephaly, midfacial hypoplasia, deep-set eyes, prominent ears). Single photon emission computed tomography (SPECT) demonstrates reduced blood flow in the frontal lobes. The disorder is associated with a deletion in the 15q11q13 chromosomal region.

■ DELUSIONS AND PSYCHOSIS

Delusions are false beliefs based on incorrect inference; they may be accompanied by hallucinations. Manifestations of *psychosis* include positive symptoms (delusions, hallucinations, disorders of communication, abnormal motor activity) and negative symptoms (avolition, poverty of thought content, affective flattening) (Table 3–3).

Delusions are typically persecutory, involving beliefs of personal endangerment, surveillance by others, being followed or harassed, being cheated, or being plotted or conspired against. In some cases, the delusion may have a specific limited content such as the belief that someone has been replaced by an impostor (Capgras syndrome), delusions of infestation, the belief that one has an exact double (heutoscopy, doppelganger), or the belief that an influential person is secretly in love with one (erotomania, de Clerambault syndrome).

Schneiderian first-rank symptoms are a specific subset of symptoms originally described by Schneider as indicative of schizophrenia but since demonstrated to be present in psychotic mood disorders and neurologic diseases with psychosis. First-rank

TABLE 3–3. **Symptoms of psychosis**

Positive symptoms
  Delusions
    Othello syndrome (jealousy)
    Parasitosis
    Lycanthropy (werewolfism)
    de Clerambault's syndrome (erotomania)
    Incubus syndrome (phantom lover)
    Picture sign (individuals on television are present in the house)
    Koro (one's genitals are withdrawing into the abdomen)
    Dorian Gray syndrome (one is not aging)
    Capgras syndrome (others have been replaced by impostors)
    Fregoli's syndrome (a persecutor assumes the appearance of others)
    Intermetamorphosis syndrome (those around look like one's
      enemies)
    Heutoscopy (seeing oneself)
    Doppelganger (one has a double)
  Hallucinations
    Auditory
    Visual
    Tactile
    Olfactory
    Gustatory
    Somatic
  Language and communication changes
    Circumstantiality
    Tangentiality
    Derailment
    Loose associations (loss of goal)
  Abnormal motor activity
    Catatonia
    Grossly disorganized behavior
Negative symptoms
  Poverty of speech output
  Poverty of thought content
  Affective flattening
  Avolition/apathy

(continued)

TABLE 3–3. **Symptoms of psychosis** *(continued)*

Schneiderian first-rank symptoms
  Thought insertion
  Thought withdrawal
  Thought broadcasting
  Hearing one's thoughts spoken aloud
  Hearing voices arguing about or discussing one
  Hearing voice's comment on one's actions
  Delusional interpretation of one's perceptions
  Experiencing bodily sensations as if imposed from outside
  Experiencing affect as if imposed and controlled from outside
  Experiencing impulses as if imposed and controlled from outside
  Experiencing motor actions as if imposed and controlled from outside

---

symptoms include thought insertion, thought withdrawal, thought broadcasting, hearing one's thoughts spoken aloud, hearing voices discussing or commenting on one's actions, and experiencing one's bodily sensations, affect, impulses, or motor actions imposed from the outside. Delusions may be mood congruent, with grandiose beliefs of personal power or wealth in mania and nihilistic beliefs of personal inadequacy, guilt, disease, or death in depression. Mood-incongruent delusions are beliefs whose content is not indicative of either mania or depression.

Delusions are associated with limbic system dysfunction, and most diseases with delusional manifestations involve the temporal lobes or subcortical limbic system structures (Table 3–4).

Delusions respond to treatment with traditional neuroleptic agents or with novel antipsychotic medications (Chapter 14). Anticonvulsants ameliorate delusions when the false beliefs occur as part of an ictal event. A combination of antidepressant and antipsychotic treatment provides the most efficacious relief of mood-congruent depressive delusions, and combined antimanic and antipsychotic therapy ameliorates mood-congruent delusions in mania.

TABLE 3–4.	**Brain disorders with delusions**

Schizophrenia
Epilepsy (especially temporal lobe epilepsy)
Alzheimer's disease
Frontotemporal dementias (e.g., Pick's disease)
Cortical Lewy body disease
Huntington's disease
Parkinson's disease after treatment with dopaminergic agents
Idiopathic basal ganglia calcification
Posttraumatic encephalopathy
Viral encephalitis (especially herpes encephalitis)
Creutzfeldt-Jakob disease
Stroke (particularly involving the temporal lobes, such as in patients with Wernicke's aphasia)
Vascular dementia
Multiple sclerosis
Metachromatic leukodystrophy
Adrenoleukodystrophy
Brain tumors (particularly involving the temporal lobes)
Vitamin B_{12} deficiency
G_{M2} gangliosidosis
Neuronal ceroid lipofuscinosis
Mitochondrial encephalopathy

■ HALLUCINATIONS AND ILLUSIONS

Hallucinations are sensory experiences occurring without stimulation of the relevant sensory organ. In psychotic disorders, hallucinations are considered veridical events, whereas hallucinations are recognized as false perceptions in nonpsychotic syndromes. *Illusions* are misperceptions of external events. Hallucinations and illusions commonly occur in the same disorders. Hallucinations may involve any sensory modality: visual, auditory, gustatory, olfactory, and tactile. Hallucinations may be formed and recognizable (e.g., visual hallucinations of people or animals), or they may be simple and unformed (e.g., visual hallucinations consisting of spots, lights, or colors).

Visual hallucinations occur with lesions of the eyes, optic nerves, geniculocalcarine projections, occipital cortex, or temporal lobes (Table 3–5). Blindness due to cataracts, retinal, or macular disease may be associated with formed or unformed hallucinations. *Charles Bonnet syndrome* is characterized by ocular disease and hallucinosis in elderly persons. Hallucinations may occur with destructive lesions of the hemispheres *("release" hallucinations)* or as ictal events in the course of focal epileptic seizures. *Ictal hallucinations* are usually brief and stereotyped, and they are associated with other seizure manifestations (e.g., head and eye turning, interruption of consciousness), whereas hallucinations occurring with destructive lesions are typically more prolonged and variable and occur within a visual field defect. Destructive lesions may produce either formed or unformed hallucinations; ictal hallucinations are unformed when the focus is in the occipital lobe and formed when it is in the temporal lobe. Formed hallucinations occurring with temporal lobe seizures may be visual memories.

Peduncular hallucinosis is a unique hallucinatory syndrome occurring with midbrain lesions and consisting of a sleep disturbance and well-formed, often Lilliputian hallucinations that occur in the evening and have an amusing quality. *Migraine* headaches may be preceded by visual hallucinations; these are usually nonformed scintillations or semiformed fortification spectra but may be fully formed visual images. *Narcolepsy* is a brain stem dysregulation syndrome manifested by the tetrad of visual hallucinations, sleep attacks, cataplexy, and sleep paralysis. Hallucinations in narcolepsy occur on falling asleep (hypnagogic) or on awakening (hypnopompic). Visual hallucinations may also occur with degenerative brain disease and are particularly common in cortical Lewy body disease and in Parkinson's disease after initiation of dopaminergic treatment.

Auditory hallucinations occur with acquired deafness, brain stem lesions, temporal lobe seizures, or with any psychotic disor-

TABLE 3–5.   Differential diagnosis of visual hallucinations

Ocular disorders
   Macular degeneration
   Cataracts
   Enucleation
Optic nerve and tract disorders
   Multiple sclerosis
   Ischemia
   Compression by a mass
Midbrain lesions (peduncular hallucinosis)
   Stroke
   Tumors
Geniculocalcarine radiation lesions ("release" hallucinations)
   Stroke
   Tumors
   Multiple sclerosis
Occipital or temporal cortex
   Stroke
   Tumors
   Seizures
Other conditions
   Migraine
   Narcolepsy
   Alzheimer's disease
   Cortical Lewy body disease
   Parkinson's disease after dopaminergic treatment
   Drug intoxication or withdrawal
   Metabolic encephalopathies
   Schizophrenia
   Depression or mania with mood-congruent hallucinations

der (Table 3–4). Musical hallucinations are common in elderly individuals with partial deafness. *Gustatory hallucinations* are most common with seizures affecting the medial temporal (uncus) region. Ictal hallucinations are treated with anticonvulsants (Chapter 14); nonictal hallucinations have no specific treatment but may respond to antipsychotic agents.

■ ANXIETY

Anxiety has emotional and cognitive, motoric, and autonomic manifestations. *Emotional and cognitive disturbances* include excessive and unjustified apprehension, feelings of foreboding, and thoughts of impending doom. Patients are irritable, feel keyed up, and have difficulty concentrating. *Motor abnormalities* include tremor (typically a high-frequency, low-amplitude tremor of the hands), an exaggerated startle response, and restlessness with frequent shifting of posture, pacing, and fidgeting. Facial expression conveys the patient's excessive concern. *Autonomic disturbances* of anxiety include sweating, palpitations, gastrointestinal distress (nausea, diarrhea), shortness of breath, dry mouth, light-headedness, and frequent urination.

Several types of anxiety disorders are recognized: panic disorder (discrete periods of anxiety that are unexpected and unpredictable), agoraphobia (excessive fear of situations from which escape would be difficult or embarrassing), social phobia (exaggerated fear of situations that expose one to scrutiny by others), specific phobia (abnormal fears of objects or situations such as insects, snakes, blood, heights, or elevators), and generalized anxiety disorder (anxiety about two or more life circumstances occurring on most days of a 6-month period). Posttraumatic stress disorder (PTSD) is an anxiety disorder that occurs in individuals who have experienced unusually severe psychological stress. It is characterized by reexperiencing the traumatic event, avoiding stimuli associated with the trauma or a generalized reduction in emotional responsiveness, and heightened arousal (difficulty sleeping, irritability, hypervigilance, exaggerated startle response, and autonomic symptoms when exposed to events that resemble the traumatic event) (Table 13–5). Some classifications of anxiety include obsessive-compulsive disorder (OCD); this syndrome is discussed below.

The neuroanatomic structures and neurophysiologic mechanisms involved in anxiety have not been completely determined. Focal lesions associated with anxiety usually involve the limbic system, and more right-sided than left-sided lesions have been reported. Neurologic conditions associated with anxiety include stroke, epilepsy (particularly temporal lobe epilepsy), Parkinson's disease, migraine, multiple sclerosis, encephalitis, and posttraumatic and postconcussive syndromes. Parkinsonian patients with the "on-off" syndrome (abrupt fluctuations of mobility after long-term treatment with levodopa) often experience increased anxiety during off periods in concert with decreased mobility. Anxiety has been reported most commonly with poststroke depression in patients with lesions of the left frontal cortex and in patients with right temporal lobe lesions. Anxiety often accompanies hypoxia, hypoglycemia, hyperthyroidism, and mitral valve prolapse. It can be induced by amphetamines, cocaine, sympathomimetic agents, caffeine, lidocaine, procaine, and alcohol and drug withdrawal.

Anxiety disorders respond to treatment with behavioral therapy and to pharmacotherapy with benzodiazepines, buspirone, β-adrenergic-receptor blocking agents (e.g., propranolol), tricyclic antidepressants, and monoamine oxidase inhibitors (Chapter 14).

■ OBSESSIVE-COMPULSIVE DISORDER AND OTHER REPETITIVE BEHAVIORS

OCD is characterized by recurrent, intrusive ego-dystonic thoughts, impulses, or images *(obsessions)* and ritualistic behaviors (hand washing, checking), mental acts (counting, repeating words), and obligatory ego-dystonic motor behaviors (touching, echoing the actions of others) *(compulsions)*. The individual recognizes that the thoughts and actions are excessive and does not experience them as imposed from without (i.e., the person is not delusional).

Positron-emission tomographic (PET) studies of patients with idiopathic OCD reveal increased metabolic activity in the orbitofrontal cortex and caudate nuclei. Patients with OCD also have increased levels of somatostatin in their cerebrospinal fluid, more neurologic soft signs than age-matched control subjects, subtle neuropsychological deficits, and nonspecific EEG abnormalities.

OCD also occurs in patients with disorders of the caudate nuclei or globus pallidus and in patients with frontal lobe degenerations (Table 3–6). Frontal lobe degenerative diseases are frequently accompanied by atrophy of the caudate nuclei, and OCD in these conditions may reflect the subcortical abnormalities. All patients with disorders associated with OCD (idiopathic and neurologic) exhibit dysfunction of the orbitofrontal-subcortical circuit, whose member structures include the orbitofrontal cortex, caudate nucleus, globus pallidus, and thalamus. Decreased pallidal inhibition of the thalamus with resultant thalamocortical excitation

TABLE 3–6. **Etiologies of obsessive-compulsive symptoms**

Site of dysfunction	Etiology
Orbitofrontal cortex	Idiopathic obsessive-compulsive disorder
Caudate nucleus	Frontal lobe degenerations with caudate atrophy
	Pick's disease
	Frontal lobe degeneration without specific histologic changes
	Huntington's disease
	Neuroacanthocytosis
	Parkinson's disease
	Tourette syndrome
	Anoxic-ischemic caudate lesions
	Sydenham's chorea
Globus pallidus	Postencephalitic parkinsonism
	Manganese intoxication
	Carbon monoxide toxicity
	Anoxic-ischemic lesions
	Progressive supranuclear palsy

is a common pathophysiologic alteration that is associated with most etiologies of OCD. Compulsive behavior may also be produced by amphetamines and other psychostimulants and by levodopa.

OCD responds to treatment with behavioral therapy and to pharmacologic intervention with serotonergic agents (Chapter 14). Neurosurgery is useful for treatment-resistant patients; anterior capsulotomy has produced the highest rate of improvement.

A variety of other repetitive behaviors occur in patients with brain dysfunction (Table 3–7). The relationship of these repetitious activities to OCD has not been fully determined; a trial of medications useful in OCD is warranted when the behavior is of disabling severity.

■ PERSONALITY ALTERATIONS

A variety of personality alterations occur in neurologic disease. No widely accepted systematic classification of personality changes associated with specific neurologic disorders or accompanying lesions in restricted brain regions has been developed. The most important diagnostic feature is a *change* from the individual's previous personality characteristics. There is often an exaggeration of previous personality traits plus new behavioral patterns associated with regional brain dysfunction. Irritability, apathy, and exaggerated emotionality are behavioral alterations common to many neurologic disorders.

Personality changes with frontal lobe dysfunction (Chapter 4) are well known, but many other types of personality alterations are observed in patients with neurologic disorders. Table 3–8 lists the most commonly reported personality traits in patients with neurologic diseases. Most types of personality change are refractory to pharmacologic treatment; aggressive or agitated behavior may respond to neuroleptics, trazodone, carbamazepine, valproate, benzodiazepines, or antidepressants.

TABLE 3–7. **Repetitive behaviors observed in patients with brain dysfunction**

Repetitive behavior	Description	Etiologies
Echolalia	Repetition of what is heard	TS, DD, advanced dementia
Palilalia	Repetition of one's own words	TS, DD, advanced dementia, basal ganglia disorders
Logoclonia	Repetition of the final syllable of words	Advanced dementia
Coprolalia	Cursing	TS, neuroacanthocytosis, basal ganglia disorders
Echopraxia	Imitating the actions of others	TS, hyperekplexias
Copropraxia	Obscene gesturing	TS, basal ganglia disorders
Carphologia	Handling, picking	Advanced dementia
Trichotillo-mania	Pulling out one's hair	TS, idiopathic
Lip biting	Self-inflicted perioral bites	Lesch-Nyhan syndrome, neuroacanthocytosis
Self-injurious behavior	Cutting oneself, drug overdose, or other wounding	Epilepsy, TS, personality disorders
Stereotypy	Repetitive non-goal-directed movements	Psychosis (idiopathic or with neurologic disease), Rett's syndrome, autism
Mannerisms	Repetitive goal-directed movements	Psychosis (idiopathic or with neurologic disease), autism
Exhibitionism	Removing clothing	TS, idiopathic paraphilia, Huntington's disease
Hypermetamor-phosis	Exploration of environ-mental stimuli	Klüver-Bucy syndrome with bilateral temporal lobe lesions
Perseveration	Repetition of the last or a recently performed motor act	Frontal lobe disorders; dementia
Oculogyric crises	Forced eye deviation	Postencephalitic parkinson-ism, neuroleptic-induced parkinsonism

Note. DD = developmental delay. TS = Tourette syndrome.

TABLE 3–8. **Personality alterations in neurologic disorders**

Personality change	Neurologic disorder
Apathy	Medial frontal lesions; basal ganglia disorders; thalamic lesions; vascular dementia; HIV encephalopathy
Disinhibition	Orbitofrontal lesions (degenerations, tumors, trauma); caudate disorders
Irritability	Orbitofrontal lesions; caudate disorders (particularly Huntington's disease)
Explosive	Posttraumatic encephalopathy, DD, Huntington's disease
Indifference	Alzheimer's disease
Placidity	Klüver-Bucy syndrome with bilateral temporal lobe dysfunction
Suspiciousness	Epilepsy; Huntington's disease; focal lesions with Wernicke's aphasia or pure word deafness
Temporal lobe epilepsy personality	Temporal lobe epilepsy (characterized by hypergraphia, interpersonal viscosity and stickiness, circumstantiality in spontaneous speech, hyperreligiosity, and hyposexuality)
Alexithymia	Right-hemisphere lesions
Schizoid behavior	Childhood-onset right-brain lesions

Note. DD = developmental delay. HIV = human immunodeficiency virus.

■ DISSOCIATIVE DISORDERS

Dissociative disorders are characterized by lapses of memory (psychogenic amnesia), periodic unrecallable behavior (psychogenic fugue and multiple personality disorder), feelings of being detached from one's body (depersonalization), and feelings of unreality or of being disengaged from one's environment (derealization, trance state). Patients with psychogenic amnesia, fugue, and multiple personality have intact, integrated behavior during the period that cannot be recollected later. In fugue states, the individual is confused about his or her identity or assumes a new identity; in multiple personality disorder, the individual has two or more distinct personalities that alternately take control of the person's behavior. *Psychogenic amnesia* must be distinguished from *transient global amnesia.* In the former condition, learning is intact at a time when the patient is unable to recall past information, there is a disproportionate involvement of personal information, and remote recall is more impaired than learning of new information. In the latter condition, the patient has an ongoing amnesia during the episode and does not learn new information; recent memory is more affected that remote recall. *Psychogenic fugues* must be distinguished from "twilight states" and poriomania (aimless wandering) occurring with *complex partial seizures.* Patients with the former condition exhibit integrated behavior during the episode, whereas individuals with the latter condition are usually in confusional states and may have other seizure-related phenomena (automatisms, lip smacking, incontinence, generalized seizures).

Depersonalization and *derealization* occur in a variety of neurologic disorders, including partial complex seizures, migraine, postconcussive states, encephalitis, and acute confusional states accompanying toxic-metabolic disorders. Depersonalization and derealization may also occur in the course of anxiety attacks.

■ ALTERED SEXUAL BEHAVIOR AND PARAPHILIC DISORDERS

Sexual activity may be increased, decreased, or altered in orientation by neuropsychiatric illnesses. Diminished libido with decreased interest in sexual behavior is the most common alteration. Hyposexuality occurs in epilepsy, stroke (particularly after right-hemisphere injury), Parkinson's disease and most parkinsonian syndromes, Alzheimer's disease, and multiple sclerosis. Reduced sexual behavior follows injury or surgery to the posterior hypothalamus. Many medications reduce libido or interfere with erectile or ejaculatory function and result in decreased sexual function.

Increased libido with heightened interest in sexual activity is more unusual in neuropsychiatric disorders. It has been reported in conjunction with secondary mania (discussed above), right thalamic injury without mania, orbitofrontal dysfunction, septal injury (after placement of ventriculoperitoneal shunts), bilateral caudate lesions, and the *Klüver-Bucy syndrome*. The latter consists of hypersexuality, emotional placidity, hypermetamorphosis (compulsory exploration of high-stimulus items in the environment), hyperorality (a tendency to place items in the mouth), and dietary changes. Disorders with bilateral medial temporal lobe involvement produce the Klüver-Bucy syndrome (Table 3–9); it is most commonly associated with herpes encephalitis. A few classes of drugs—stimulants, testosterone-containing agents, and dopaminergic agents—may increase libido.

TABLE 3–9.   **Etiologies of the Klüver-Bucy syndrome**

Postencephalitic syndromes after herpes encephalitis

Trauma

Alzheimer's disease

Pick's disease

Frontotemporal degeneration without Pick's cells

Adrenoleukodystrophy

Delayed, postanoxic leukoencephalopathy

Bilateral temporal lobe stroke

Postpartum coagulopathy with stroke

Status epilepticus with bilateral temporal lobe foci

Bilateral temporal lobectomy (for control of seizures)

Postictal state with bilateral temporal lobe foci

Amygdalotomy (bilateral)

Posttraumatic encephalopathy

Paraneoplastic limbic encephalitis

Hypoglycemia

Toxoplasmosis

Paraphilic disorders are characterized by intense sexual urges or sexually arousing fantasies involving nonhuman objects, suffering or humiliation of oneself or one's partner, and children or nonconsenting adults. Examples of paraphilias include exhibitionism (exposing one's genitals), fetishism (nonliving objects), frotteurism (touching or rubbing against a nonconsenting person), pedophilia (prepubescent children), sexual masochism (being humiliated, beaten, or bound), sexual sadism (psychological or physical suffering of a victim), transvestic fetishism (cross-dressing), and voyeurism (observing an unsuspecting person who is naked, disrobing, or engaging in sexual activity). Many rarer types of paraphilias involving uncommon stimuli that induce sexual arousal have been described. Paraphilic behavior has been reported in conjunction with temporal lobe epilepsy, postencephalitic parkinsonism, frontal lobe disorders, Huntington's disease, multiple sclerosis, and Tourette syndrome.

■ REFERENCES AND RECOMMENDED READING

Altemus M, Pigott T, L'Heureux F, et al: CSF somatostatin in obsessive-compulsive disorder. Am J Psychiatry 150:460–464, 1993

American Psychiatric Association: Diagnostic and Statistical Manual of Mental Disorders, 4th Edition. Washington, DC, American Psychiatric Association, 1994

Baxter LR, Schwartz JM, Bergman KS, et al: Caudate glucose metabolic rate changes with both drug and behavior therapy for obsessive-compulsive disorder. Arch Gen Psychiatry 49:681–689, 1992

Cummings JL: Clinical Neuropsychiatry. New York, Grune & Stratton, 1985

Cummings JL: Depression and Parkinson's disease: a review. Am J Psychiatry 149:443–454, 1992

Cummings JL: Frontal-subcortical circuits and human behavior. Arch Neurol 50:873–880, 1993

Cummings JL, Miller BL: Visual hallucinations. Clinical occurrence and use in differential diagnosis. West J Med 146:46–51, 1987

Cummings JL, Petry S, Dian L, et al: Organic personality disorders in dementia syndromes: an inventory approach. J Neuropsychiatry Clin Neurosci 2:261–267, 1990

Gorman DG, Cummings JL: Organic delusional syndrome. Semin Neurol 10:229–238, 1990

Joffe RT, Lippert GP, Gray TA, et al: Mood disorder and multiple sclerosis. Arch Neurol 44:376–378, 1987

Lilly R, Cummings JL, Benson DF, et al: The human Klüver-Bucy syndrome. Neurology 33:1141–1145, 1983

Mascari MJ, Nicholls RD, Levin J, et al: Prader-Willi syndrome and Angelman syndrome, in Static Encephalopathies of Infancy and Childhood. Edited by Miller G, Ramer JC. New York, Raven, 1992, pp 177–195

Mayberg HS, Starkstein SE, Sadzot B, et al: Selective hypometabolism in the inferior frontal lobe in depressed patients with Parkinson's disease. Ann Neurol 28:57–64, 1990

Mayberg HS, Starkstein SE, Peyser CE, et al: Paralimbic frontal lobe hypometabolism in depression associated with Huntington's disease. Neurology 42:1791–1797, 1992

Mendez MF, Cummings JL, Benson DF: Depression in epilepsy. Significance and phenomenology. Arch Neurol 43:766–770, 1986

Miller BL, Cummings JL, McIntyre H, et al: Hypersexuality or altered sexual preference following brain injury. J Neurol Neurosurg Psychiatry 49:867–873, 1986

Nissenbaum H, Quinne NP, Brown RG, et al: Mood swings associated with the "on-off" phenomenon in Parkinson's disease. Psychol Med 17:899–904, 1987

Robinson RG, Starkstein SE: Current research in affective disorders following stroke. J Neuropsychiatry Clin Neurosci 2:1–14, 1990

Starkstein SE, Robinson RG (eds): Depression in Neurologic Disease. Baltimore, MD, Johns Hopkins University Press, 1993

Taylor MA: The Neuropsychiatric Guide to Modern Everyday Psychiatry. New York, Free Press, 1993

Trimble MR: Biological Psychiatry. New York, Wiley, 1988

Trimble MR: Behavior and personality disturbances, in Neurology in Clinical Practice. Edited by Bradley WG, Daroff RB, Fenichel GM, et al. Boston, MA, Butterworth-Heinemann, 1991, pp 81–100

FRONTAL LOBE SYNDROMES

The frontal lobes are the largest lobes of the brain, comprising almost one-third of the total cortical surface area. They are among the latest evolutionary additions to the brain and are larger in humans than in any other species. They complete myelination late in the maturation cycle and become functional in the final phases of ontogenetic development. The frontal lobes receive information about the external environment from sensory association cortices and information about the individual's emotional state and internal milieu from the limbic system and hypothalamus. They are anatomically poised to integrate environmental and emotional information and to formulate and execute an action plan. They initiate volitional activity and control the motor system, thus mediating the action of the individual on the environment. The frontal lobes bestow many of the uniquely human characteristics of behavior, and diseases of the frontal lobe are among the most dramatic in neuropsychiatry. Frontal lobe anatomy is described in Chapter 2.

■ FRONTAL LOBE SYNDROMES

Frontal lobes are divided in the motor cortex adjacent to the Rolandic fissure, the premotor cortex anterior to the motor cortex, and the prefrontal cortex comprising the region anterior to the premotor areas. Contralateral weakness, brisk reflexes, and Babinski signs occur with lesions of the motor strip; Broca's aphasia and executive aprosodia (Chapter 5) follow lesions of the left and right premotor areas, respectively; and alterations in cognition, demeanor, and mood are associated with prefrontal dysfunction.

Prefrontal cortex mediates complex human behavior, and three major behavioral syndromes associated with prefrontal dysfunction have been identified. The three critical prefrontal regions are the dorsolateral prefrontal area, the orbitofrontal area, and the anterior cingulate area. In addition, these three regions are the origins of three distinct frontal-subcortical circuits that mediate circuit-specific behaviors (Chapter 2). The marker behaviors of dysfunction of these regions and of the associated subcortical circuits are executive dysfunction (the dorsolateral prefrontal syndrome), disinhibition (the orbitofrontal syndrome), and apathy (the medial frontal/anterior cingulate syndrome).

Most lesions or diseases affecting the frontal lobes involve multiple frontal lobe regions, and combinations of the three principal syndromes are the rule in clinical practice. Patients exhibit a spectrum of performance failures from mild to severe. Moreover, patients rarely fail all tests of functions ascribed to a particular region; it is the overall pattern of successes and failures that leads to recognition of a frontal lobe syndrome rather than performance on any individual test. Finally, tests of frontal lobe function may be disrupted by lesions outside the frontal lobes and frontal-subcortical circuits, and it is only when failure occurs in the absence of dysfunction in other areas that the performance deficits can be correlated with frontal lobe or frontal systems dysfunction (for example, reduced verbal fluency can be attributed to prefrontal dysfunction only in patients with intact language function).

DORSOLATERAL PREFRONTAL SYNDROME

Dorsolateral prefrontal disorders are marked by executive dysfunction characterized by poor strategies including impaired planning when copying constructions and when organizing material to be remembered, impaired set shifting in response to changing task contingencies, abnormalities of motor programming, compromised attention, and environmental dependency (Table 4–1).

Compromised learning strategies are most evident on tests of new learning where the patient is asked to learn a list of words. Patients with dorsolateral prefrontal dysfunction do not organize the information efficiently and thus have difficulty with spontaneous recall after a delay. However, they usually learn a substantial

TABLE 4–1. **Frontal lobe syndromes and their assessment**

Frontal region	Characteristic abnormality	Assessment
Dorsolateral prefrontal	Reduced verbal fluency	Verbal fluency: letter or category naming
	Reduced nonverbal fluency	Design fluency test[a]
	Poor set shifting	Wisconsin Card Sorting Test; Trails B
	Impaired abstraction	Similarities, differences, proverb interpretation, cognitive estimates
	Poor judgment	Evaluate insight and plans[a]
	Poor response inhibition	Stroop Color-Word Interference Test
	Reduced spontaneous recall	Delayed recall test[a] (Rey Auditory Verbal Learning Test or California Verbal Learning Test)
	Poor memory organization	California Verbal Learning Test
	Poor drawing strategies	Copy of complex figure (Rey-Osterrieth or Taylor Complex Figures)
	Reduced divided attention	Consonant trigrams
	Reduced sustained attention	Cancellation tests
	Perseveration on sequential motor tasks	Alternating programs, reciprocal programs, multiple loops, serial hand sequences[a]
Orbitofrontal	Disinhibition	Rating scale assessment; impulsive, tactless behavior
	Anosmia	Tests of olfaction
Anterior cingulate	Apathy	Rating scale assessment; reduced motivation, interest, and activity

(continued)

TABLE 4–1. **Frontal lobe syndromes and their assessment**
(continued)

Frontal region	Characteristic abnormality	Assessment
Frontal eye fields	Reduced contralateral gaze	Sustained gaze deviation
Inferior pre-motor (left)	Broca's aphasia	Language assessment (Boston Diagnostic Aphasia Examination or the Western Aphasia Battery)
Inferior pre-motor (right)	Executive aprosodia	Listen to patient's spontaneous vocal inflection, and ask patient to imitate various inflections modeled by the examiner (happiness, sadness, surprise, anger)
Primary motor cortex	Contralateral hemiparesis	Contralateral weakness involving the extensors of the arm and the flexors of the leg, contralateral hyperreflexia with an extensor plantar response (Babinski sign)

Note. Representative types of tests are listed; most tests are described in the text.
[a]These tests are particularly useful for bedside testing.

amount of the information, and this can be demonstrated by providing them with an opportunity to choose the previously learned words from a multiple-choice list. The patients exhibit the retrieval deficit syndrome, as evidenced by poor recall and preserved recognition memory. Amnestic syndromes characterized by poor recall and poor recognition occur with frontal lobe dysfunction only when deeply placed lesions affect the fornix as it courses through the frontal lobe on its trajectory from hippocampus to hypothalamus or when the lesion involves the basal forebrain, producing an interruption of cholinergic innervation of the hippocampus.

Impaired search of semantic memory and manipulation of knowledge are evident on tasks of verbal fluency in which the patient is asked to name as many members of a specific category (e.g., animals or words beginning with a specific letter of the alphabet) as possible in 1 minute. Patients with left-sided dorsolateral prefrontal dysfunction have disproportionate difficulty with this task. A normal performance is 18 animals per minute; fewer than 12 animals recalled in 1 minute is definitely abnormal. An approximately equivalent nonverbal fluency task sensitive to right-sided dorsolateral prefrontal dysfunction requires that the patient generate as many figures that are composed of four lines of equal length as possible in 1 minute. Each line must intersect at least one other line, and the figures must not be repeated. A normal performance is 10 figures per minute; fewer than 8 is abnormal. Figure 4–1 provides examples of normal and abnormal performances on the nonverbal fluency test. The test is particularly difficult for patients with right dorsolateral prefrontal dysfunction.

Poor strategies for copying tasks are demonstrated by asking patients to copy a complex figure and observing their approach. They typically have a segmented approach, reproducing individual elements and failing to organize their drawing around the principal figure elements. Overemphasis of the high-stimulus areas of the figure is also common.

Poor set shifting is demonstrated by tasks such as Trails B and the Wisconsin Card Sorting Test, which require the patient to flexibly shift from one cognitive set to another. Several types of abnormalities may be observed on these tests: patients may be excessively slow, they may lose the set prematurely, or they may perseverate, repeating their previous responses.

Motor programming tasks assess the patient's ability to execute sequential motor acts. Examples of alternating programs (alternating between square and pointed figures) and multiple loops are shown in Figures 4–2 and 4–3. Reciprocal programs require the patient to alternate performances with the examiner. For example, the patient is asked to tap twice each time the examiner taps once

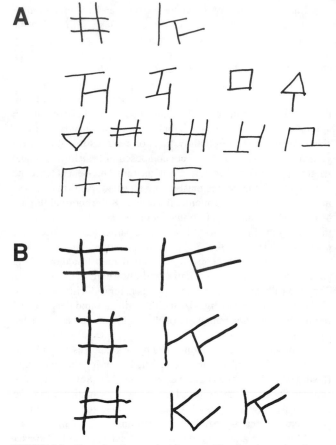

FIGURE 4–1. Examples of a normal performance *(A)* and an abnormal performance *(B)* on the design fluency test. The patient who fails the task is unable to generate a normal number of designs and produces stereotyped figures. In each case, two sample figures (comprised of four lines of equal length with each line touching at least one other line) are the first two figures and were provided by the examiner; the remaining figures were produced by the patient. The patient had a degenerative frontal lobe syndrome.

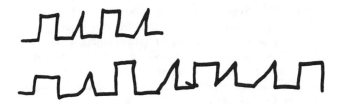

FIGURE 4–2. Example of abnormal alternating programs. The examiner's model is shown on the *top line;* the patient's attempt to reproduce the model is shown on the *bottom line.* Perseveration is evident in the patient's attempt to copy and extend the examiner's model. The patient had a frontal lobe degenerative disorder.

and to tap once each time the examiner taps twice. In the go–no go test, which is a further elaboration of this task, the patient is asked to tap once each time the examiner taps once and to withhold any response when the examiner taps twice. This test requires that the patient inhibit a response.

Another example of a motor programming test is performance of serial hand sequences with verbal guidance (e.g., having the patient say aloud "fist, slap, cut" while executing the corresponding hand postures). Patients with dorsolateral prefrontal dysfunc-

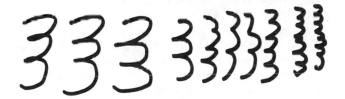

FIGURE 4–3. Examples of abnormal performance on the multiple loop test. The examiner's models are the first three figures on the *left;* the patient's abnormal copies are on the *right.* Perseveration is evident as the patient tries to reproduce the examiner's model figures. The patient had a clinical syndrome consistent with a frontal degenerative disease.

tion have difficulty with verbal mediation of motor behavior and manifest verbal-manual dissociation, saying one sequence while executing another. Tests of motor programming evaluate the patient's ability to perform a sequence of actions; impersistence with failure to continue the required acts, perseveration with repetition of a previous response, or failure to verbally guide motor behavior may be observed.

Compromised attention is also characteristic of patients with dorsolateral prefrontal dysfunction. They may fail elementary tests of attention such as digit span or continuous performance tasks. The former requires the patient to repeat a series of digits read aloud by the examiner (normally, patients can repeat a series of at least five digits). The latter tests the patient's ability to sustain his or her attention over time; the patient is asked to signal each time the letter *A* occurs in a series of letters read aloud by the examiner. The test continues for at least 1 minute. Lapses of attention result in errors of omission. Some patients perform these elementary tests satisfactorily but fail more complex attentional tests such as mental control (repeating the months of the year in reverse order), response inhibition (as required by the Stroop test, in which the patient must read aloud the color in which a word is printed rather than the word itself), and divided attention (such as consonant trigrams, which require the patient to memorize three letters, then count backward serially, and then repeat the three letters).

Environmental dependency is evident with frontal lobe dysfunction and may reflect attentional and motivational abnormalities. The patient's attention is inappropriately dominated by environmental stimuli. For example, when patients with dorsolateral prefrontal dysfunction are asked to set the hands of a clock to read 11:10, they may put one hand on the 11 and one on the 10. The 10 is an environmental stimulus that attracts their attention and creates an erroneous behavior.

Mood changes are common with dorsolateral prefrontal lesions. Approximately 60% of patients with acute lesions in this area have depressive symptoms. Half of the patients have a major depressive episode, and half have a minor or dysthymic-type depression. Anxiety frequently accompanies the depression in patients with lesions affecting the frontal cortex. Studies with positron-emission tomography (PET) demonstrate that patients with idiopathic depression have reduced metabolism in this region compared with nondepressed patients. Obsessive-compulsive disorder (OCD) occurs in patients with degenerative diseases affecting the dorsolateral convexity (e.g., frontal lobe degenerations such as Pick's disease); these behaviors may be physiologically related to the alterations in subcortical structures that accompany many frontal degenerative syndromes. Delusions and hallucinations are uncommon with dorsolateral prefrontal dysfunction unless other brain regions are also affected.

If the lesion or disease affecting the dorsolateral convexity extends sufficiently posterior to affect the premotor area of the left hemisphere, Broca's aphasia is present (discussed in Chapter 5). A similarly placed lesion in the right hemisphere produces an aprosodia, as evidenced by diminished inflection of spontaneous speech. A lesion affecting the motor strip produces a contralateral hemiparesis with increased muscle stretch reflexes and an extensor response to stimulation of the plantar surface of the foot (Babinski's sign). The weakness is most marked in the extensor muscles of the arm (e.g., deltoid, triceps, brachioradialis; resulting in a tendency to keep the arm flexed) and in the flexor muscles of the leg (iliopsoas, hamstrings, peroneals; producing an extensor posture of the leg). When the frontal eye field is affected unilaterally, the patient has ipsilateral gaze deviation or gaze preference. Prefrontal lesions can also produce contralateral neglect, usually manifested by a lack of action directed into the neglected space (hemi-inintention).

ORBITOFRONTAL SYNDROME

The orbitofrontal syndrome is the most dramatic of all frontal disorders. Individuals with previously normal behavior are transformed by the prefrontal lesion. The predominant behavioral change is disinhibition; lack of restraint is manifested in a myriad of ways. Patients ignore social conventions and exhibit undue familiarity, talking to strangers and touching or fondling others without permission. They are tactless in conversation and may make uncivil or lewd remarks. They are impulsive, responding immediately and unpredictably to changing environmental circumstances. They lack conscientiousness and fail to complete assigned tasks. They are unconcerned about the consequences of their behavior and may engage in activities that endanger themselves or others. Risk assessment is poor. They have been labeled "pseudopsychopathic" because of the similarity of some of their behaviors to those of individuals with antisocial personality disorders.

Mood alterations also accompany the orbitofrontal syndrome. Lability and irritability are the most common changes. Patients rapidly shift from happiness (often a vacuous ebullient euphoria) to anger or sadness. Mood changes are rarely sustained, and anger can often be relieved by redirecting the patient's attention to some new activity. Hypomania or mania may accompany orbitofrontal dysfunction.

Studies of brain metabolism have shown abnormalities affecting this region in a variety of behavioral disorders. Orbitofrontal glucose metabolism is increased in patients with idiopathic OCD. Metabolism in this region is decreased in patients with Parkinson's disease and depression and in patients with Huntington's disease and depression compared with nondepressed individuals with these movement disorders.

The elementary neurologic examination of patients with the orbitofrontal syndrome reveals few abnormalities. Olfaction may be impaired because of the proximity of the olfactory nerves, bulbs, and tracts to the inferior orbitofrontal surface. Intellectual changes are notably absent in patients with lesions limited to the orbitofrontal cortex. Language, memory, and visuospatial skills are unaffected, although distractibility, irritability, and failure to cooperate may compromise test performance.

MEDIAL FRONTAL SYNDROME

The medial frontal syndrome is marked by apathy. The apathy has emotional, cognitive, and motor dimensions. *Emotionally,* the apathetic individual is unmotivated to initiate new tasks; there is a disinterest in establishing or accomplishing goals. There is little that excites or stimulates the individual; mood changes may include an emotional emptiness or "eutonia," an unrealistic feeling of well-being. *Cognitively,* the apathetic individual fails to formulate or implement plans and activities; there is a loss of generative thought. Slowing of cognition may be evident. The patient with a left unilateral lesion may have transcortical motor aphasia (Chapter 5) characterized by transient mutism recovering to a nonfluent verbal output with preserved repetition and comprehension. Contralateral neglect may occur in the period immediately after onset of an acute cingulate lesion. *Motorically,* apathetic individuals do not engage in activities. They may sit for long periods without participating in functions. In the most extreme form of apathy, the syndrome of *akinetic mutism,* the individual is awake but motionless and mute. Such individuals will eat if fed, and they may occasionally move or speak briefly. They are not paralyzed, and the syndrome must be distinguished from locked-in syndrome and catatonia. Stimulation of the cingulate in humans or nonhuman primates produces vocalization, autonomic and visceral responses, and repetitive motor behaviors.

Frontal lobe disorders producing the apathetic syndrome involve the medial frontal region, particularly the anterior cingulate cortex. The syndrome of akinetic mutism occurs transiently in patients with unilateral medial frontal lesions; permanent akinetic mutism is observed with bilateral medial frontal dysfunction. Apathy also occurs in patients with lesions of the caudate nucleus, globus pallidus, and thalamus; these are member structures of the medial frontal-subcortical circuit.

Relatively few abnormalities of neuropsychological function or of the elementary neurologic examination accompany medial frontal lobe lesions. A grasp reflex is commonly present and may be one of three types: contact grasp, elicited by placing the examiner's hand in the palm of the patient's hand; traction grasp, elicited by slowly withdrawing the examiner's hand from the patient's hand along the palmar surface; and magnetic grasp, elicited by touching the back of the patient's hand and producing a following response as the examiner lifts his or her hands vertically. Neuropsychologically, patients with medial frontal lesions may exhibit abnormalities on the go–no go test, echoing the examiner's actions instead of following instructions. (For example, when the patient is asked to hold up two fingers when the examiner holds up one finger and to make no response when the examiner holds up two fingers, the patient exhibits echopraxia, reproducing the examiner's movements.)

Cingulectomy or cingulotomy ameliorates chronic pain, OCD, depression, anxiety, and aggression. The wide range of disorders affected by cingulate interruptions suggests that the cingulate participates in many behaviors, perhaps by amplifying associated emotional intensity.

FRONTAL LOBE DYSFUNCTION ASSOCIATED WITH WHITE MATTER INJURY

In addition to the three principal prefrontal syndromes described above, alterations attributable to disorders of the frontal white matter also occur. These alterations may be seen with demyelinating (e.g., multiple sclerosis), ischemic (e.g, Binswanger's disease), or compression (e.g., normal-pressure hydrocephalus) syndromes. Gait abnormalities commonly accompany disorders involving the frontal white matter. The most typical gait change has been called "lower-half parkinsonism" and is comprised of reduced step height and limited stride length. A foot grasp reflex may be present, producing a magnetic-type sticking of the foot to the floor. Poor balance and retropulsion may be evident. Urinary and occasionally fecal incontinence may also be present.

TABLE 4–2. **Disorders of the frontal lobes**

Class of disorder and examples	Frontal region affected
Degenerative	
Pick's disease	Prefrontal
FLD without Pick bodies	Prefrontal
ALS with dementia	Prefrontal
Alzheimer's disease	Prefrontal (severe changes late)
Cortical Lewy body disease	Diffuse
Vascular	
Anterior cerebral artery occlusion	Medial frontal
Anterior cerebral artery aneurysm rupture	Orbitofrontal
Middle cerebral artery occlusion	Lateral convexity
Binswanger's disease	Periventricular
Traumatic	
Closed head injury	Orbitofrontal contusion, diffuse axonal injury to white matter fibers
Penetrating injury	Local and diffuse
Demyelinating	
Multiple sclerosis	White matter (especially periventricular)
Metachromatic leukodystrophy	White matter (begins frontally)
Marchiafava-Bignami disease	Corpus callosum (anteriorly)
Neoplastic	
Meningioma	
Subfrontal	Orbitofrontal
Convexity	Lateral convexity
Falcine	Medial frontal
Glioblastoma, oligodendroglioma, metastasis	Local with diffuse edema
Infectious	
Creutzfeldt-Jakob disease	Focal onset with rapid spread
Syphilis	Prefrontal
Herpes encephalitis	Orbitofrontal and temporal
Inflammatory	
Systemic lupus erythematosus and other inflammatory disorders	Diffuse

Note. ALS = amyotrophic lateral sclerosis. FLD = frontal lobe degeneration.

■ DISEASES OF THE FRONTAL LOBES

Table 4–2 lists the major disorders that affect the frontal lobes and notes the frontal regions most likely to be affected by each process. These disorders are discussed in more detail in other chapters of this volume.

■ REFERENCES AND RECOMMENDED READING

Alexander GE, DeLong MR, Strick PL. Parallel organization of functionally segregated circuits linking basal ganglia and cortex. Annu Rev Neurosci 9:357–381, 1986

Ballantine HT, Bouckoms AJ, Thomas EK, et al: Treatment of psychiatric illness by stereotactic cingulotomy. Biol Psychiatry 22:807–817, 1987

Cummings JL: Frontal-subcortical circuits and human behavior. Arch Neurol 50:873–880, 1993

Cummings JL, Coffey EC: Neurobiological basis of behavior, in Textbook of Geriatric Neuropsychiatry. Edited by Coffey EC, Cummings JL. Washington, DC, American Psychiatric Press, 1994, pp 71–96

Damasio AR, Anderson SW: The frontal lobes, in Clinical Neuropsychology, 3rd Edition. Edited by Heilman KM, Valenstein E. New York, Oxford University Press, 1993, pp 409–460

Eslinger PJ, Damasio AR: Severe disturbance of higher cognition after bilateral frontal lobe ablation: patient EVR. Neurology 35:1731–1741, 1985

Fuster JM: The Prefrontal Cortex, 2nd Edition. New York, Raven, 1989

Lhermitte F, Pillon B, Serdaru M: Human autonomy and the frontal lobes, part I: imitation and utilization behavior: a neuropsychological study of 75 patients. Ann Neurol 19:326–334, 1986

Lhermitte F: Human autonomy and the frontal lobes, part II. Patient behavior in complex and social situations: the "environmental dependency syndrome." Ann Neurol 19:335–343, 1986

Macmillan MB: A wonderful journey through skull and brains: the travels of Mr. Gage's tamping iron. Brain Cogn 5:67–107, 1986

Mattson AJ, Levin HS: Frontal lobe dysfunction following closed head injury. J Nerv Ment Dis 178:282–291, 1990

McClelland RJ: Psychosocial sequelae of head injury—anatomy of a relationship. Br J Psychiatry 153:141–146, 1988

Mesulam M-M: Patterns in behavioral neuroanatomy: association areas, the limbic system, and hemispheric specialization, in Principles of Behavioral Neurology. Edited by Mesulam M-M. Philadelphia, PA, FA Davis, 1985, pp 1–70

Miller BL, Cummings JL, Villaneuva-Meyer J, et al: Frontal lobe degeneration: clinical, neuropsychological, and SPECT characteristics. Neurology 41:1374–1382, 1991

Novoa O, Ardila A: Linguistic abilities in patients with prefrontal damage. Brain Cogn 30:206–225, 1987

Price BH, Daffner KR, Stowe RM, et al: The comportmental and learning disabilities of early frontal lobe damage. Brain 113:1383–1393, 1990

Ron MA: Psychiatric manifestations of frontal lobe tumours. Br J Psychiatry 155:735–738, 1989

Stuss DT, Benson DF: The Frontal Lobes. New York, Raven, 1986

Weinberger DR: A connectionist approach to the prefrontal cortex. J Neuropsychiatry Clin Neurosci 5:241–253, 1993

APHASIA AND RELATED SYNDROMES

This chapter addresses disorders of verbal output including aphasia, aprosodia, amusia, dysarthria, mutism, and reiterative speech disturbances such as stuttering, echolalia, and palilalia. In addition, neurobehavioral disorders occurring with left-hemisphere dysfunction and frequently observed in patients with aphasia (apraxia, acalculia, Gerstmann syndrome) are also described. The clinical features, anatomic correlates, and appropriate assessments and interventions appropriate for aphasias and related conditions are presented. Fundamental to understanding aphasia and related syndromes is information regarding handedness, hemispheric specialization, and cerebral dominance. These concepts are discussed before describing the aphasic disorders and other syndromes associated with left-hemisphere dysfunction.

5

■ HEMISPHERIC SPECIALIZATION, CEREBRAL DOMINANCE, AND HANDEDNESS

A uniquely well-developed aspect of human brain organization is hemispheric specialization. This refers to the asymmetric mediation of neuropsychological and behavioral functions. Cerebral dominance refers to the corresponding principle that one hemisphere is usually superior to the other with regard to a specific task and is dominant for that function. Neither hemisphere is dominant for all functions; in general, the left hemisphere is dominant for language-related tasks, and the right hemisphere is superior for visuospatial tasks. The left brain, however, has the capacity to mediate some visuospatial functions, and the right brain has at least rudimentary language skills. Table 5–1 provides an overview of tasks with known asymmetric hemispheric demands.

TABLE 5–1.	**Skills and abilities mediated asymmetrically by the two hemispheres**

Left hemisphere

 Propositional speech

 Language comprehension

 Naming

 Reading

 Writing

 Praxis (skilled movements)

 Calculation

Right hemisphere

 Facial discrimination

 Facial recognition

 Depth perception

 Receptive affective prosody

 Executive affective prosody

 Music

 Constructional abilities

 Mental rotation of shapes

A few anatomic asymmetries between the hemispheres have been identified. These include asymmetric Sylvian fissures (more horizontal on the left, more vertical on the right), larger occipital horn of the left lateral ventricle, longer left hemisphere, wider right frontal lobe, increased left cortical area in Broca's area on the left, larger left pulvinar, and asymmetric decussation (fibers descending from the left brain cross first) in the cerebral medulla. The anatomic differences are relatively modest compared with the marked functional differences between the hemispheres.

Handedness is related to cerebral dominance and is the most readily available means of assessing cerebral dominance for language. Ninety-nine percent of right-handed individuals have left cerebral dominance for language. Among left-handers, approximately 70% are also left-brain dominant for language, 15% have language skills mediated primarily by the right hemisphere, and 15% have bilateral representation of language.

■ APHASIA

Aphasia refers to an impairment in linguistic communication produced by brain dysfunction. It must be distinguished from other disorders of verbal output such as dysarthria, mutism, and the abnormal language production of patients with formal thought disorders. Nine principal aphasia syndromes are recognized (Table 5–2); each of these has unique characteristics and occurs with brain dysfunction in specific brain regions. The three principal features that differentiate the aphasias are fluency of verbal output, ability to comprehend spoken language, and ability to repeat phrases stated by the examiner. The rules guiding localization provided here apply to right-handed adults. Left-handed individuals often have atypical patterns of hemispheric dominance and manifest less predictable clinical syndromes associated with brain lesions. Children often have nonfluent verbal output regardless of lesion location.

Fluency refers to the flow of spontaneous speech. Aphasias are either fluent or nonfluent. *Fluent aphasias* are characterized by normal or increased rate of speech, preserved speech melody, normal phrase length, preserved grammatical constructions (minor grammatical errors may occur), empty speech with impoverished information content, and the presence of paraphasic errors. Paraphasias may be phonemic (substitution of a single phoneme or syllable), verbal (substitution of one word for another), or neologistic (production of novel words that have no meaning). Wernicke's, anomic, conduction, thalamic, and transcortical sensory aphasias are all fluent. Fluent aphasias occur with post-Rolandic lesions sparing the anterior hemispheric regions.

Nonfluent aphasias feature sparse, effortful verbal output with reduced amount of speech, short phrase length, abnormal

TABLE 5–2. **Characteristics of the aphasia syndromes**

Syndrome	Fluency	Comprehension	Repetition	Localization in left hemisphere
Wernicke's	Fluent	Impaired	Impaired	Posterior superior temporal
Transcortical sensory	Fluent	Impaired	Intact	Angular gyrus
Thalamic[a]	Fluent	Impaired	Intact	Thalamus
Conduction	Fluent	Intact	Impaired	Arcuate fasciculus
Anomic	Fluent	Intact	Intact	Anterior temporal; angular gyrus
Broca's	Nonfluent	Intact	Impaired	Inferior frontal
Transcortical motor	Nonfluent	Intact	Intact	Medial frontal or superior to Broca's area
Global	Nonfluent	Impaired	Impaired	Wernicke's and Broca's areas
Mixed transcortical	Nonfluent	Impaired	Intact	Lesions of transcortical motor and transcortical sensory aphasias

[a]Thalamic aphasia is usually distinguished from transcortical sensory aphasia associated with cortical lesions by the onset with mutism, co-occurring dysarthria, and prominent hemiparesis.

prosody (rhythm and melody of speech), and agrammatism (loss of short grammatical "functor" words such as *to, in, then,* etc.). There is relative preservation of the informational content of speech, and there are few paraphasic errors; dysarthria may be present. Global, Broca's, transcortical motor, and mixed transcortical aphasias are nonfluent. Nonfluent aphasias are associated with lesions that involve the pre-Rolandic brain regions.

Comprehension of spoken language is assessed by asking the patient to follow commands, decipher yes-and-no questions, and respond to sentences with complex grammatical constructions. Commands frequently request a pointing response ("point to the ceiling," "point to the door and then to the ceiling," "point to your nose, your wrist, and your chin"). Yes-and-no questions assess the patient's ability to understand language content and grammar ("Are the lights in this room on?" "Do you put your shoes on before your socks?" "Do you have your lunch before your breakfast?"). More complex questions can also be formulated, such as "Is my wife's brother a man or a woman?" and "If a lion and a tiger were in a fight and the lion was killed by the tiger, which animal was dead?" Comprehension is impaired (not necessarily completely absent) in patients with lesions that involve Wernicke's area and the angular gyrus region and is preserved in patients with lesions that spare these areas.

Repetition is evaluated by asking the patient to repeat words, phrases, and sentences. The examination begins by asking the patient to repeat single words to ensure that the patient understands the task ("say after me 'boy,'" "say 'basketball player'"). Then the patient is asked to repeat phrases ("no ifs, ands, or buts") and sentences ("she went home early," "the truck rolled over the stone bridge," "the quick brown fox jumped over the lazy dog"). Repetition is impaired in patients with lesions involving the structures abutting the Sylvian fissure (Wernicke's, conduction, Broca's, global aphasias) and is spared in patients with lesions removed from the peri-Sylvian area (anomic, transcortical motor, transcortical sensory, mixed transcortical, and thalamic aphasias).

Naming is impaired in all aphasic syndromes. Paraphasic naming errors may be observed in fluent aphasic disorders. Errors in *writing* generally reflect the disturbances observed in spontaneous speech. *Reading comprehension* is impaired in most patients with reduced auditory comprehension; *reading aloud* is impaired in Wernicke's, Broca's, conduction, global, and mixed transcortical aphasias. Singing, automatic speech (reciting the alphabet or counting), and cursing are preserved in many aphasias, even those with severe verbal output disturbances.

Aphasias occur with a wide variety of neurologic disorders that affect the left hemisphere including stroke, tumors, trauma, infections (herpes encephalitis, Creutzfeldt-Jakob disease, abscesses), and degenerative diseases such as Alzheimer's disease, frontotemporal dementias, and primary progressive aphasia.

In addition to the bedside tests described above, formal aphasia evaluations can be performed by speech and language therapists or neuropsychologists. Magnetic resonance imaging (MRI) is the optimal technique for demonstrating focal brain lesions associated with aphasia. Computed tomography (CT) will reveal most aphasia-producing lesions. Positron-emission tomography (PET) and single photon emission computed tomography (SPECT) usually reveal areas of functional impairment that are larger than the structural lesions demonstrated by MRI and CT in aphasic patients.

Patients with acute aphasias secondary to stroke or trauma may be helped by speech and language therapy and should be referred to a speech therapist for evaluation and construction of a treatment program.

■ ALEXIAS AND AGRAPHIAS

Alexia refers to an acquired inability to read and *agraphia* to an acquired inability to write. These terms are not applicable to illiterate individuals who never developed significant reading and writing skills. Three alexias are recognized. *Alexia with agraphia* occurs with lesions of the left angular gyrus or the left posterior inferior temporal lobe. The patients cannot read or write and are not aided by spelling the words aloud. They perform as if truly illiterate. *Alexia without agraphia* is observed with lesions of the medial left occipital cortex and the splenium of the corpus callosum or lesions of the left lateral geniculate body and splenium of the corpus callosum. The patients can often understand written words by spelling the words aloud and recognizing the word from the letters they hear. Alexia without agraphia is an example of a *disconnection syndrome:* the right occipital lobe perceives the information to be read, but the signal cannot be transferred to the left hemisphere because of the lesion of the corpus callosum. The left and right hemispheres are disconnected. Conduction aphasia (discussed above) and sympathetic and callosal apraxias (discussed below) are other examples of disconnection syndromes. *Frontal alexia* occurs with lesions of the left frontal lobe, and most patients with frontal alexia have Broca's aphasia. The reading deficit of frontal alexia involves an inability to name individual letters and disturbed comprehension of written language contingent on grammatical constructions and accurate interpretation of functor words (e.g., "put the red circle *on top of* the blue square").

Agraphia occurs in several circumstances including linguistic, spatial, apractic, and motor disturbances. *Linguistic agraphias* occur in all aphasias, as a part of the Gerstmann syndrome and the angular gyrus syndrome (discussed below), and in the syndrome of alexia with agraphia (discussed above). In aphasia, the written output mirrors the patient's spontaneous verbalizations. Anterior lesions result in nonfluent agraphia with agrammatism, whereas posterior lesions are associated with fluent agraphias characterized by written paraphasias and relative preservation of syntax.

Spatial agraphias are most common with lesions of the posterior right hemisphere. The patient neglects the left side of the page, there is a gradually enlarging margin on the left, letters are omitted or repeated, and the spacing of the words and letters is uneven.

Apractic agraphia is a disorder of orthography that is manifest in spite of normal sensorimotor function and intact letter and word knowledge. Patients can type normally, establishing the integrity of their linguistic and motor functions. Manual writing, including copying letters produced by others, is disrupted. Lesions of the left superior parietal region have been associated with the syndrome.

Mechanical agraphias accompany motor disorders that affect the limbs and are described in patients with parkinsonism (micrographia), choreas, dystonic disorders (writer's cramp), and cerebellar syndromes. Action tremors disrupt writing, and some tremors are elicited virtually only by the act of writing (primary writing tremors).

■ APROSODIA

Prosody refers to the melodic, intonational, and inflectional aspects of speech. Much of the informational content of verbalization is conveyed through prosody rather than through its propositional (verbal) components. Prosody plays a role in dialect (regional variations in word pronunciation), linguistic communication (e.g., differentiating a statement from a question), conveyance of attitude (e.g., sarcasm), and portraying emotion (e.g., sadness, anger). Prosody has executive and receptive aspects. Executive prosody refers to the patient's ability to produce prosodically accurate utterances; receptive prosody refers to the patient's ability to comprehend the prosodic aspects of another's speech (e.g., deduce the individual's emotional state). Linguistic prosody is affected by left-hemisphere and basal ganglia lesions, whereas affective and emotional prosody is impaired by right-hemisphere and basal ganglia lesions. Gesture is usually reduced in patients with affective dysprosody, and pantomime is impaired in patients with linguistic dysprosody. Damage to the region of the right hemisphere equivalent to Broca's area produces an executive affective aprosodia; injury to the right-hemisphere equivalent of Wernicke's area produces a receptive affective aprosodia.

Executive prosody is assessed by asking the patient to state a neutral sentence (e.g., "I'm going to the store") with inflections denoting anger, happiness, surprise, and sadness. Prosodic comprehension is evaluated by asking the patient to identify which emotion is present as the examiner says the sentence with each of the four different inflections.

Patients with executive aprosodia have great difficulty communicating their feelings, and their emotional distress may be underestimated. Children who sustain right-hemisphere injuries depriving them of the ability to communicate their own emotions or to comprehend the emotions of others may develop an asocial or schizoid demeanor.

■ AMUSIA

The amusias encompass syndromes characterized by loss of ability to sing (executive amusia) and to recognize or appreciate features of heard music (receptive or sensory amusia). Several brain regions are involved in the processing of musical stimuli. Lesions of the right temporal lobe impair appreciation of timbre, pitch, and intensity as well as tonal memory. Lesions of the right frontal lobe impair tonal processing. In contrast, left anterior hemispheric lesions tend to produce rhythm disturbances. Changes in musical abilities resemble those involving prosody: right temporal lesions produce primarily receptive musical and prosodic deficits, whereas right and left frontal injuries impair different aspects of executive musical and prosodic abilities. The right temporal lobe has a greater role in processing unfamiliar melodic sequences, and the left temporal lobe has a greater role in processing familiar sequences.

■ DYSARTHRIA

Dysarthria refers to impairment of the motor aspects of speech. Dysarthria results from loss of speed, coordination, or strength, producing abnormalities of speech articulation, phonation, or timing. Flaccid, spastic, ataxic, hypokinetic, hyperkinetic, and dystonic dysarthrias are recognized. *Flaccid dysarthrias* result from lower motor neuron, peripheral nerve, and muscular disorders and are characterized by a breathy, hypernasal sound quality with imprecise consonants. *Spastic dysarthrias* feature slow speech, strained-strangled voicing, and a monotone execution. Spastic dysarthrias occur with upper motor neuron disease and are associated with an exaggerated gag reflex, brisk muscle stretch reflexes, and pseudobulbar palsy. *Ataxic dysarthrias* include abnormal rhythm and timing of speech with abnormal sound stress patterns. They occur with diseases of the cerebellum and of the cerebellar tracts in the midbrain. *Hypokinetic dysarthrias* occur in parkinsonian syndromes and evidence reduced speech volume, reduced syllable stress, variable rate, and monotone output. Festination of speech (speaking with increasing rapidity) may occur. *Hyperkinetic* and *dystonic dysarthrias* are present in choreiform and dystonic disorders. They are notable for distorted sounds, inappropriate silences, respiratory irregularities, loudness variations, imprecise consonants, and slow rate. Dystonic dysarthrias have a strained-strangled speech quality. Dysphagia may accompany any of the dysarthrias and can be life threatening if aspiration occurs. Dysarthria may improve with speech therapy, and patients should be referred to a speech therapist for evaluation and treatment.

■ MUTISM

Mutism is the inability or unwillingness to speak, resulting in an absence or marked paucity of verbal output. Mutism usually refers to a complete or nearly complete absence of speech and nonverbal utterances. Mutism has a wide differential diagnosis, occurring in both neurologic and psychiatric disorders (Table 5–3).

Assessment of the mute patient must include a careful review of the neurologic and psychiatric history if available, as well as a thorough examination to detect evidence of focal neurologic dysfunction, catatonia, previous psychiatric treatment (e.g., tardive dyskinesia), or trauma. An Amytal interview may be helpful in some cases, particularly if a conversion reaction with mutism is suspected.

TABLE 5–3. **Differential diagnosis of mutism**

Psychiatric conditions

    Depression with catatonia

    Schizophrenia with catatonia

    Conversion disorder

Developmental conditions

    Selective mutism (e.g., mute only while at school)

    Absence of speech development (developmental delay, autism, deafness)

Neurologic disorders

    Acute phase of a nonfluent aphasia (see Table 5–1)

    Pseudobulbar palsy

    Acute phase of aphemia[a]

    Akinetic mutism

    Frontal lobe syndromes with marked abulia

    Postictal state after a generalized or partial seizure

    Herpes encephalitis

    Posttraumatic encephalopathy

Medical conditions

    Drug or alcohol intoxication

    Neuroleptic effect

    Metabolic encephalopathies (delirium)

    Hypothyroidism

---

[a]Aphemia is a syndrome of acute mutism followed by recovery to a hypophonic, breathy verbal output without aphasia; it is produced by a small lesion of Broca's area.

■ REITERATIVE SPEECH DISTURBANCES

Reiterative speech disturbances include stuttering, palilalia, echolalia, logoclonia, and perseveration. In addition, there are more complex repetitive disorders in which the patient repeats the same story again and again. Stuttering may be congenital or acquired. *Acquired stuttering* occurs with lesions of either hemisphere that involve the basal ganglia, frontal white matter, internal capsule, or external capsule. Stuttering may occur transiently in the course of recovery from aphasia and is also observed in basal ganglia disorders including Parkinson's disease. *Stuttering* involves repetition of the initial or an internal phoneme of a word. Patients with acquired stuttering have less frustration and grimacing than congenital stutterers. Other speech characteristics of stutterers include increased pause time, syllable prolongations, fast speech rate, and aprosodia. *Palilalia* refers to repetition of spontaneous utterances. It is manifest by repetition of the final phrase or last few words of a phrase (e.g., "I had eggs for breakfast, for breakfast, for breakfast"). It occurs in advanced stages of cortical dementias and in basal ganglia disorders. *Echolalia* is a syndrome featuring repetition of words and phrases that the patient hears from others (e.g., when greeted with "Hello, Mr. Brown" the patient may echo "Hello, Mr. Brown"). Echolalia occurs in patients with advanced cortical dementias, basal ganglia disorders, Tourette syndrome, mental retardation syndromes, and schizophrenia. *Logoclonia* is the term applied to repetitions limited to the final phoneme or two of a word (e.g., "Methodist Episcopal-copal-copal" or "hopping hippopotamus-amus-amus"). Logoclonia is particularly prominent in general paresis resulting from syphilitic encephalitis but can occur in patients who exhibit palilalia or echolalia. *Verbal perseveration,* which occurs most often in patients with fluent aphasia, is marked by the frequent reappearance of the same word in the patient's spontaneous speech. The *gramophone syndrome* is a disorder characterized by the repetition of a greeting or story. Each time the story is told, it is repeated in the same way regardless of whether the listener has heard it before. The syndrome occurs in frontotemporal dementias such as Pick's disease. The speech of schizophrenic patients is often characterized by the tendency to return to the same themes, but these discussions lack the rigid stereotypy of the gramophone syndrome.

■ APRAXIA

Three varieties of apraxia are recognized: limb-kinetic apraxia, ideomotor apraxia, and ideational apraxia. *Limb-kinetic apraxia* refers to the loss of dexterity and coordination of distal limb movements that cannot be accounted for by weakness or sensory loss. The impairment is evident in pantomime, imitation, and use of objects. It occurs contralateral to a hemispheric lesion.

Ideomotor apraxia refers to the inability to perform learned movement on command when the disturbance cannot be attributed to abnormalities of strength, coordination, sensory loss, or impaired comprehension. The defect is most obvious when pantomiming the use of objects (e.g., comb, toothbrush, lipstick, hammer, saw); however, it remains after the movement has been demonstrated by the examiner and the patient attempts to imitate the movement and may be evident even when the patient tries to use the object itself. Errors include abnormal sequencing of movement with perseveration of components of the movements, poor positioning of the limb with regard to the imagined object during pantomime, and impaired execution of the object-related movement.

Three types of ideomotor apraxia are recognized (Table 5–4). Parietal apraxia occurs with lesions of the inferior parietal region and underlying fibers of the arcuate fasciculus. Both limbs are apraxic, and the patient usually has conduction aphasia; typically there is no associated hemiparesis. Sympathetic apraxia is a syndrome comprised of apraxia of the left limbs in a patient with a right hemiparesis and Broca's aphasia. It occurs with lesions of the left frontal lobe. Callosal apraxia is characterized by apraxia of the

86

TABLE 5–4.   Characteristics of ideomotor apraxia

Type of apraxia	Lesion location	Apraxic limbs	Hemi-paresis	Aphasia
Ideomotor	Inferior parietal, arcuate fasciculus	Right and left	None	Conduc-tion
Sympathetic	Frontal lobe	Left	Right	Broca's
Callosal	Anterior callosal fibers	Left	None	None

left limbs. There is no aphasia or hemiparesis. The corresponding lesion is in the fibers of the anterior corpus callosum. Most patients with limb apraxia will also evidence buccal-lingual apraxia with difficulty executing oral and facial movements on command (e.g., "stick out your tongue," "blow out a match," "sniff a flower," "cough"). These apraxic syndromes are less predictable in left-handed individuals than in right-handed ones; left-handers are right dominant for praxis regardless of which hemisphere is dominant for language. Apraxia in right-handed individuals is almost always associated with a left-hemisphere lesion, but only about half of aphasic patients exhibit apraxia, suggesting that the right hemisphere compensates more readily for apraxia than for aphasia.

Ideational apraxia is a syndrome that features loss of the ability to pantomime the execution of an act that requires multiple steps to complete. For example, patients cannot demonstrate how they would fold a letter, place it in an envelope, seal it, place a stamp, and address the envelope. Pantomiming of other complex acts is similarly compromised (e.g., filling and lighting a pipe, filling a pitcher and pouring a glass of liquid). This unusual disorder occurs in patients with diffuse brain injuries and dementia.

■ ACALCULIA

Three types of acalculia have been described. The first occurs with lesions of the posterior left hemisphere that produce fluent aphasia and paraphasic errors. When the paraphasic intrusions affect numbers, the patient substitutes one number for another, making accurate computation impossible. The second occurs with lesions of the angular gyrus region and is a true anarithmetria with disruption of primary calculation concepts (addition, subtraction, division, multiplication). The third is observed in patients with lesions of the posterior right hemisphere and reflects compromised spatial abilities, disrupting proper alignment of numbers and subverting multiple-digit manipulations.

■ GERSTMANN AND ANGULAR GYRUS SYNDROMES

Gerstmann syndrome consists of agraphia, acalculia, right-left disorientation, and finger agnosia. Many patients have a mild constructional disturbance. Agraphia and acalculia are demonstrated easily with tests of writing and arithmetic. Right-left disorientation may be subtle and should be assessed by asking the patient to touch his or her own right and left limbs, to touch his or her right or left side with the opposite limb, and finally to indicate which is the clinician's right and left as the clinician faces the patient. The last test requires the patient to make a mental reversal of right and left. Finger agnosia, if severe, can be shown by asking the patient to name his or her own fingers or to indicate fingers named by the examiner. If the disturbance is more subtle, it can be demonstrated by asking the patient to show on one hand the finger equivalent to that touched by the examiner on the other hand held out of the patient's sight or by asking the patient to state how many fingers are between two touched by the examiner while the patient's eyes are closed. Gerstmann syndrome reliably indicates the presence of a left angular gyrus lesion when all elements of the syndrome are simultaneously present. Individually, the components of the syndrome can be seen with lesions of other brain regions and do not imply the presence of a lesion of the angular gyrus.

Angular gyrus syndrome occurs with lesions of the left angular gyrus; the lesions are generally larger than those producing Gerstmann syndrome. Angular gyrus syndrome includes all elements of the Gerstmann syndrome plus a constructional disturbance, alexia, anomia, parietal-type ideomotor apraxia, and verbal memory disturbance. The syndrome may be mistaken for Alzheimer's disease because there are multiple cognitive abnormalities and no motor deficits.

■ REFERENCES AND RECOMMENDED READING

Alexander MP, Fischer RS, Friedman R: Lesion localization in apractic agraphia. Arch Neurol 49:246–251, 1992

Altshuler LL, Cummings JL, Mills MJ: Mutism: differential diagnosis and report of 22 cases. Am J Psychiatry 143:1409–1414, 1986

Ardila A, Rosselli M: Spatial agraphia. Brain Cogn 22:137–147, 1993

Bell WL, Davis DL, Morgan-Fisher A, et al: Acquired aprosodia in children. J Child Neurol 5:19–26, 1990

Benson DF: Aphasia, in Clinical Neuropsychology, 3rd Edition. Edited by Heilman KM, Valenstein E. New York, Oxford University Press, 1993, pp 17–36

Blonder LX, Bowers D, Heilman KM: The role of the right hemisphere in emotional communication. Brain 114:1115–1127, 1991

Cancelliare AEB, Kertesz A: Lesion localization in acquired deficits of emotional expression and comprehension. Brain Cogn 13:133–147, 1990

Damasio A: Signs of aphasia, in Acquired Aphasia, 2nd Edition. Edited by Sarno MT. New York, Academic Press, 1991, pp 27–43

Damasio H: Neuroanatomical correlates of the aphasias, in Acquired Aphasia, 2nd Edition. Edited by Sarno MT. New York, Academic Press, 1991, pp 45–71

Darby DG: Sensory aprosodia: a clinical clue to lesions of the inferior division of the right middle cerebral artery? Neurology 43:567–572, 1993

Darley FL, Aronson AE, Brown JR: Motor Speech Disorders. Philadelphia, PA, WB Saunders, 1975

Gardner H, Winner E, Rehak A: Artistry and aphasia, in Acquired Aphasia, 2nd Edition. Edited by Sarno MT. New York, Academic Press, 1991, pp 373–404

Goodglass H, Kaplan E: The Assessment of Aphasia and Related Disorders. Philadelphia, PA, Lea & Febiger, 1976

Graff-Radford NR, Welsh K, Godersky J: Callosal apraxia. Neurology 37:100–105, 1987

Heilman KM, Rothi LJG: Apraxia, in Clinical Neuropsychology, 3rd Edition. Edited by Heilman KM, Valenstein E. New York, Oxford University Press, 1993, pp 141–163

Kertesz A, Ferro JM: Lesion size and location in ideomotor apraxia. Brain 107:921–933, 1984

Kolb B, Whishaw IQ: Fundamentals of Human Neuropsychology, 3rd Edition. New York, WH Freeman, 1990

Ludlow CL, Rosenberg J, Salazar A, et al: Site of penetrating brain lesions causing chronic acquired stuttering. Ann Neurol 22:60–66, 1987

McCarthy RA, Warrington EK: Cognitive Neuropsychology. New York, Academic Press, 1990

Mozaz MJ: Ideational and ideomotor apraxia: a qualitative analysis. Behavioural Neurology 5:11–17, 1992

Rosselli M, Ardila A: Calculation deficits in patients with right and left-hemisphere damage. Neuropsychologia 27:607–617, 1989

Sandson J, Albert ML: Perseveration in behavioral neurology. Neurology 37:1736–1741, 1987

Stommel EW, Freidman RJ, Reeves AG: Alexia without agraphia associated with spleniogeniculate infarction. Neurology 41:587–588, 1991

VISUAL AND VISUOSPATIAL DISORDERS

Visuospatial function is critically important to human survival. The visuospatial environment requires constant assessment except during sleep. Perception, nonverbal memory, constructional activities, and visual recognition of places, objects, and people are all critical aspects of visuospatial function. In this chapter, the principal visuospatial disorders are discussed, the associated lesions or causative disorders are presented, and appropriate interventions are described. Table 6–1 presents a classification of the major visuospatial disturbances.

■ VISUOPERCEPTUAL DISORDERS

Perception refers to the ability to sense a stimulus regardless of whether the stimulus is recognized. Recognition of a stimulus is a sequential process that begins with perception and progresses through stages of increasing refinement. Interruption of this process at different stages results in different types of clinical deficits. Lesions of the eye or the optic nerve produce ipsilateral blindness (partial or total); lesions behind the optic chiasm result in homonymous visual field defects; pathologic changes in the inferior calcarine cortex produce achromatopsia (central color blindness); medial occipitotemporal lesions of the right hemisphere are associated with prosopagnosia (defective recognition of familiar faces) and environmental agnosia (impaired recognition of familiar places); and bilateral lesions of the medial occipitotemporal cortex or inferior longitudinal fasciculi cause visual object agnosia.

MONOCULAR BLINDNESS

Ocular disorders—including diseases of the lens (cataracts), retina, or macula—produce total or partial blindness of the involved eye.

TABLE 6–1. **Classification of visuospatial disorders**

Visuoperceptual disorders
Monocular blindness
Homonymous hemianopsia
Achromatopsia
Cortical blindness
Simultanagnosia
Balint's syndrome
Impaired depth perception

Visual discrimination disorders
Impaired matching of lines of identical angles
Impaired matching to unfamiliar faces
Discrimination (disambiguation) of embedded figures
Matching of complex visual patterns

Visual recognition disorders
Prosopagnosia
Environmental agnosia
Visual object agnosia
Color agnosia
Finger agnosia

Visuospatial attention disorders
Neglect syndromes and anosognosia
  Unilateral neglect
  Anosognosia
  Anosognosic syndromes
Symbol or figure cancellation abnormalities

Body-spatial disorientation
Dressing disturbances
  Body-garment disorientation
  Unilateral neglect
  Multiple layering
Impaired visual determination of vertical when one's body is not vertical

(continued)

TABLE 6–1.	**Classification of visuospatial disorders** *(continued)*

Impaired map reading

Impaired route finding

Constructional disorders

  Copying deficits

  Drawing abnormalities

Visuospatial cognition and memory disorders

  Visuospatial cognition deficits

    Impaired visual synthesis and organization

    Impaired mental rotation

    Impaired strategy for complex constructions

    Poor nonverbal fluency

    Defective revisualization (Charcot-Wilbrand syndrome)

  Visual memory disturbances

    Nonverbal recall and recognition disorders

    Reduplicative paramnesia

  Right-left disorientation

Likewise, diseases of the optic nerve (such as glaucoma affecting the nerve head, ischemic optic neuritis, and optic neuritis) produce unilateral blindness ipsilateral to the lesion. Pupillary responses are usually compromised in diseases of the eye and optic nerve because there is diminished light conduction, and this sign may help distinguish blindness as a manifestation of ocular or neurologic disease from feigned blindness or blindness as a manifestation of a conversion reaction. In addition, patients with conversion disorders or who are malingering have intact optokinetic nystagmus (nystagmus that is normally induced by passing a striped cloth in front of the eyes of a sighted person). Table 6–2 presents characteristics that aid in distinguishing among different types of blindness.

    Long-standing bilateral blindness may result in pendular nystagmus with spontaneous to-and-fro movements of the eyes. Visual

TABLE 6–2. **Characteristics of blindness of different etiologies**

Characteristic	Prechiasmal lesion	Cortical blindness	Blindness as a conversion symptom
Direct pupillary reaction	Absent	Present	Present
Consensual pupillary reaction	Present[a]	Present	Present
Optokinetic nystagmus	Absent	Absent	Present
Visual evoked response	Abnormal	Abnormal	Normal

[a]A consensual pupillary response is present in blindness with prechiasmal lesions when the blindness is unilateral; bilateral prechiasmal blindness would eliminate the consensual response.

hallucinations ("release" hallucinations) are not uncommon in patients with ocular disorders and may be either formed or unformed. Phosphenes (sudden flashes of light) often accompany retinal or optic nerve disease, and some patients may experience synesthesia characterized by phosphenes occurring in response to loud sounds or noises.

Visual evoked responses are slowed in patients with optic nerve disease; they offer a means of documenting the presence of disease in patients with normal fundoscopic examinations. Visual evoked potentials may be slowed even when visual acuity is measurably normal and may be useful in establishing the presence of optic nerve disease in patients with suspected multiple sclerosis.

HOMONYMOUS HEMIANOPSIA

Lesions of the optic tract, optic chiasm, geniculate nucleus of the thalamus, or the geniculocalcarine radiations produce homonymous visual-field defects. Temporal lobe lesions are associated with asymmetric (incongruent) field defects; occipital lesions cause symmetric (congruent) defects. Lesions involving the entire radiation produce homonymous hemianopsias (usually with sparing of the central few degrees of vision), whereas lesions affecting only some of the fiber tracts produce quadrantanopsias or other incomplete field defects. Pupillary responses are intact in patients with homonymous visual-field defects, and visual acuity is normal. Hallucinations are common in the period immediately after an injury to the geniculocalcarine radiations (e.g., in the first few days after a stroke) and may be unformed (lights), semiformed (tire track or herringbone patterns), or formed (complex scenes, animals, or people). The hallucinations are commonly confined to the area of the visual-field defect.

ACHROMATOPSIA

Achromatopsia refers to central color blindness. The patient loses the ability to distinguish color in the contralateral visual field. The associated lesions involve the cortex inferior to the calcarine fissure of the medial occipital lobe. There is often an associated partial hemianopsia. The color blindness is difficult to demonstrate except when it is bilateral. Color blindness is assessed with color-naming tests, tests requiring sorting of colors by shades, and Ishihara pseudoisochromatic plates.

CORTICAL BLINDNESS

Cortical or cerebral blindness occurs when bilateral lesions of the geniculocalcarine radiations or occipital cortex deprive the patient of all vision. Patients may be totally blind or may have sufficient residual vision to distinguish light from darkness and to be able to count fingers. If there is sparing of central vision, patients may be able to see minimally by moving their heads to allow exploration of the environment through a tiny retained central visual field. These patients may see very small objects better than large objects because they can see small objects as a whole in their reduced visual field but must scan large objects. Pupillary responses are intact, but optokinetic nystagmus is lost.

The most common cause of cortical blindness is occlusion of both posterior cerebral arteries with bilateral medial occipital infarction. The lesions may be demonstrated by computed tomography (CT) or magnetic resonance imaging (MRI). Cortical blindness has also occurred with diffuse cortical injuries such as anoxic insults.

Anton's syndrome consists of blindness with denial of blindness. Patients claim to see and even describe what they think they see but are inaccurate in the descriptions and can be shown to be blind. Anton's syndrome occurs most commonly in patients with cortical blindness but may also occur in patients with other types of blindness when they are in acute confusional states or develop dementia. Many patients with blindness due to bilateral posterior cerebral lesions are severely agitated even if they are unaware of their blindness.

■ SIMULTANAGNOSIA

Agnosias are recognition deficits rather than perceptual disturbances. Simultanagnosia is a misnamed exception. In this disorder, when the patients are shown two objects simultaneously, they fail to perceive one of them. For example, when shown a figure consisting of a circle and a cross, they see the circle or the cross but not both; when shown a number drawn by juxtaposing many small numbers (for example the number 2 drawn by using many little number 3s), they see the number 2 or the number 3s but not both. The neurophysiologic basis of this mysterious condition has not be determined, but it is most often attributed to an abnormality of visual attention. Simultanagnosia typically occurs in patients with bilateral parietal lobe lesions.

Simultanagnosia is often observed as part of *Balint's syndrome*. The latter consists of optic ataxia (the inability to touch objects accurately using visual guidance), sticky fixation (difficulty volitionally redirecting gaze), and simultanagnosia.

■ VISUAL DISCRIMINATION DISORDERS

Impaired visual discrimination takes many forms, and each can be demonstrated with a specific discrimination task. Discrimination abnormalities include difficulty matching lines that subtend identical angles, impaired matching of unfamiliar faces (e.g., faces with different emotional expressions or faces viewed from different angles), reduced discrimination (disambiguation) of overlapping figures, and impaired matching of complex visual patterns. These disorders are all more common with lesions of the posterior aspect of the right hemisphere than with lesions elsewhere in the brain.

■ VISUAL RECOGNITION DISORDERS

PROSOPAGNOSIA

Prosopagnosia refers to the inability to recognize familiar faces. Visual perception is intact; the patient sees normally and can describe the unrecognized face in detail. However, familiar faces, such as the faces of family members and famous people, cannot be recognized. In some cases, specific facial features (moustache, glasses of a specific type) are used to facilitate recognition, but the patient is easily fooled if someone with similar characteristics appears. When the person's voice is heard, recognition is usually immediate, demonstrating that nonvisual means of recognition and naming are intact. Tests of visual discrimination (e.g., matching faces photographed from two different angles and matching different faces with similar emotional expressions) are not necessarily compromised; facial recognition and facial discrimination are different neuropsychological capacities mediated by different processes and affected by lesions in different locations.

Bilateral medial occipital lesions are present in many reported patients with prosopagnosia, but right unilateral regions appear to be sufficient to produce the syndrome.

ENVIRONMENTAL AGNOSIA

Environmental agnosia is a clinical syndrome characterized by the inability to recognize familiar places. The patient sees normally and is able to describe the surroundings but has no sense of familiarity. Patients commonly adopt verbal strategies to compensate for the deficit; for example, they may find their homes by using the street signs and house numbers. Environmental agnosia and prosopagnosia frequently coexist. The causative lesion is in the medial occipitotemporal region of the right hemisphere.

VISUAL OBJECT AGNOSIA

Two principal types of visual object agnosia have been identified, apperceptive agnosia and associative agnosia. The two identified syndromes reflect disruption of different stages of processing of complex visual information, and variations of the syndromes are common. *Apperceptive visual agnosia* is characterized by intact visual acuity but an inability to recognize objects. Patients can distinguish shades of light intensity, identify colors, determine line orientation, exhibit depth perception, see movement, and distinguish thin from thick lines. They can negotiate their surroundings but cannot recognize, describe, or match perceived objects. They cannot draw objects they see and cannot point to objects named by the examiner. The agnosia involves all visual stimuli including faces, the environment, and objects. Variability over time is characteristic of the patients, and they often complain of fleeting or unstable vision. Apperceptive agnosia may occur as a phase of recovery from cortical blindness after anoxia, carbon monoxide poisoning, or bilateral posterior hemispheric strokes.

Associative visual agnosia features intact elementary perception and preserved ability to describe, draw, and match visual stimuli. For example, when shown an object (shoe, toothbrush, etc.), patients can draw the object and match the object with an identical one from a group of objects, but they cannot recognize the object or describe its use. When allowed to touch the object or hear any sounds the object may make (such as a bell or ring), patients immediately recognize the object and can describe it or demonstrate its use. Object recognition by touch demonstrates that the patient is not anomic and that the agnosia is modality specific, limited to the visual domain. Agnosia for faces, letters, and colors usually but not invariably accompanies the visual object recognition defect. Visual-field defects, particularly a right homonymous hemianopsia, may be present. Most patients with associative visual agnosia have diffuse cortical injury or bilateral medial occipitotemporal lesions involving the cortex or the inferior longitudinal fasciculi.

COLOR AGNOSIA

Color agnosia (also called color anomia) is present in some patients who have alexia without agraphia (Chapter 4). The patients do not have abnormalities of color naming and can name the colors appropriate to specific settings (a banana is yellow, a fire engine is red); they also can sort and match colors. They do not have color blindness. They cannot point to named colors or name colors pointed to by the examiner. The patients have lesions of the medial left occipital cortex and the splenium of the corpus callosum.

Finger agnosia, the disorder accompanying Gerstmann syndrome, is characterized by an inability to name, localize, or discriminate among fingers.

■ DISTURBANCES OF VISUOSPATIAL ATTENTION

UNILATERAL NEGLECT

Unilateral (or hemispatial) neglect refers to a lack of attention to events and actions in one-half of space. Neglect may involve all sensory modalities—visual, auditory, and somatosensory—as well as motor acts (motor neglect) and motivation. *Unilateral visual neglect* is the most commonly observed form of hemispatial neglect. In its most subtle form, the patient ignores the stimulus presented in the neglected hemifield when two visual stimuli are presented simultaneously in the visual fields. This type of neglect can be demonstrated by holding one hand in equivalent portions of each visual field while facing the patient, quickly moving the fingers of each hand, and asking the patient to point to the hand whose fingers moved (the technique of double simultaneous stimulation). The patient will perceive movement only in the nonneglected visual field.

In its more obvious form, unilateral visual neglect may be evidenced by failure to copy one-half of model objects, read one-half of words, dress one-half of the body, or shave one-half of the face. Tests for visual neglect include line bisection (the patient crosses the line in the middle of the nonneglected portion) and the line-crossing test, in which the patient is given a sheet of paper with randomly distributed lines and is asked to cross each line in the middle; only those lines in the nonneglected field will be crossed. Constructional tasks such as asking the patient to copy a figure (Figure 6–1) or draw a clock often reveal the neglect: the patient copies or draws only the nonneglected portion of the figure. Clock-drawing tests can be misleading in patients with frontal lobe syndromes and poor planning because these patients fail to properly space the figures on the clock face and may include most of the digits on one part of the clock, thus producing a drawing that superficially resembles figures produced by patients with true unilateral neglect.

Neglect may occur in the absence of a homonymous hemianopsia, and patients with homonymous field defects may learn to compensate for their visual impairment if they do not have a neglect syndrome. Neglect and visual-field defects have no obligatory relationship and must be assessed separately.

In severe forms of neglect, all types of stimuli in the affected hemiuniverse are neglected. *Somesthetic neglect* is demonstrated by touching the patient simultaneously on both sides of the body

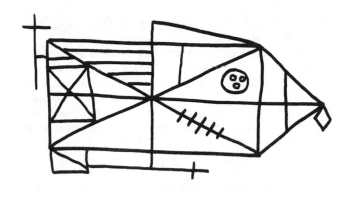

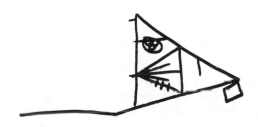

FIGURE 6-1. Rey-Osterrieth Complex Figure *(above)* and a copy of the figure made by a patient with a right parietal lobe lesion *(below)*. The copy demonstrates neglect of the left half of the figure.

and asking the patient where he or she was touched; the patient perceives only the touch on the nonneglected side of the body. *Auditory neglect* is assessed by standing behind the patient, snapping the fingers on either or both sides of the head, and asking the patient to point toward the side where a stimulus was heard. The patient points only toward the nonneglected side during double simultaneous auditory stimulation.

Sensory neglect is most severe and enduring after damage to the right parietal region, but it may occur with left parietal and subcortical lesions. Hemispatial neglect is contralateral to the side of the lesion.

Motor neglect syndromes involve action-intention disorders affecting the half of space contralateral to frontal lobe or basal ganglia lesions. The patient is aware of stimuli in the neglected hemispace (no sensory neglect is present) but produces no motor response in the neglected area. The patient may appear to have a hemiparesis because the limb with action-intention neglect is unused, but when strength and coordination are tested, they are found to be normal. The abnormality may be most evident when the patient is asked to perform movements with both arms such as extending them both or drawing circles in the air with both: the limb with action-intention neglect fails to perform normally.

ANOSOGNOSIA AND ANOSOGNOSIC SYNDROMES

Anosognosia is the clinical syndrome characterized by denial of hemiparesis. It classically occurs in patients with right parietal lesions and left unilateral neglect who deny their left hemiparesis. The extended syndrome of denial of illness may involve other types of disability such as blindness and aphasia. Risk factors for persistent anosognosia include large right-sided lesions, severe left-sided neglect, cognitive and memory deficits, apathy, and cerebral atrophy.

Variants of anosognosia include somatophrenia (denial of ownership of the paralyzed limbs), anosodiaphoria (minimization of and unconcern about the weakness without complete denial), misoplegia (hatred of the paralyzed or weak limb), personification (naming the limb and giving it an identity), and supernumerary limbs (reduplication of limbs on the neglected side). Patients with anosognosia or its variants typically have other evidence of neglect such as extinguishing stimuli on the paretic side during double simultaneous stimulation or failure to reproduce elements on the neglected side when asked to copy model figures.

SYMBOL OR FIGURE CANCELLATION ABNORMALITIES

In addition to lateralized neglect contralateral to a hemispheric lesion, some patients may have nonlateralized visual attention disturbances. These occur with frontal lobe lesions or more diffuse cerebral disorders (extensive white matter alterations) and can be demonstrated by asking the patient to survey a page with multiple letters or symbols and circle or cross out a specific target. The targets are most likely to be neglected on the side contralateral to the lesion, but targets may be missed in any part of space.

■ BODY-SPATIAL DISORIENTATION

DRESSING DISTURBANCES

Although frequently called dressing "apraxia," these abnormalities rarely meet the criteria presented in Chapter 5 for apraxia and are best regarded as special cases of visuospatial disorders. They are more closely related to constructional and visual synthesis abnormalities than to executive visuomotor abnormalities. Three types of dressing disturbances are observed in clinical practice. *Body-garment disorientation* occurs essentially exclusively with right parietal lobe lesions and consists of an inability to properly orient the limbs and trunk with respect to clothing. The patient may put on a shirt or blouse inside-out or even try to put a leg into a sleeve. The task is made particularly difficult by giving the patient a garment that is inside-out and asking him or her to correct it and put it on. *Unilateral neglect* may be manifest by dressing only one-half of the body. The patient may put only one arm (the nonneglected side) into a shirt or may comb the hair on only one-half of the head. A third type of dressing disturbance, *excessive layering* of clothes, occurs in patients with dementia and schizophrenia.

OTHER BODY-SPATIAL DISTURBANCES

Other disorders of orientation of the body within space include impaired visual determination of vertical when one's body is not vertical, impaired map reading, and impaired route finding when no map is used.

■ CONSTRUCTIONAL DISORDERS

Constructions are the best means of assessing visuospatial function in the clinic or at the bedside, and copying and drawing tests should be part of every mental status examination. A series of constructions of graded difficulty is used to assess copying skills. Begin by having the patient draw a circle; this helps him or her understand the test, experience some initial success, and engage the task. Then have the patient copy more complicated figures such as a diamond, overlapping rectangles, a cube, or more demanding models such as the Rey-Osterrieth or Taylor Complex Figures (Figure 6–2). Drawing abilities can be evaluated by asking the patient to draw a clock, a flower, and a house.

Copying tests assess both perception and executive visuomotor abilities and may be affected by occipital, parietal, or frontal lobe dysfunction of either hemisphere. Temporal lobe lesions have little effect on copying tests. Unilateral neglect implies the presence of a lesion of the contralateral hemisphere; other lesion effects are less discriminating. Occipitoparietal lesions disturb perception and figure recognition and tend to produce more profound constructional changes. Left-hemisphere lesions tend to have a greater effect on the patient's ability to reproduce the internal detail of an object, while leaving the ability to reproduce the external configuration intact. Right-sided lesions have the opposite effect, ad-

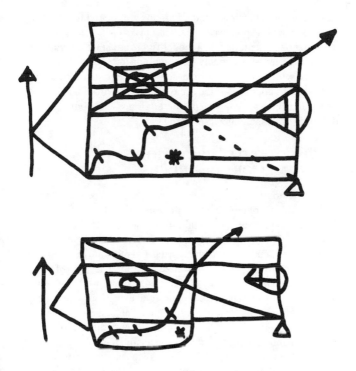

FIGURE 6–2. Taylor Complex Figure *(above)* and a copy of the figure made by a patient with a dementia syndrome and visuospatial dysfunction *(below).* The copy demonstrates distortions and omissions.

versely affecting the patient's ability to reproduce the orientation and external configuration of objects while leaving intact the execution of internal detail. Frontal lobe lesions affect the strategy used by patients to accomplish the copying task; these patients usually take a fragmented approach to the task, copying individual subsegments of the figure and overdeveloping portions of the figure that attract their attention. Patients with parietal lobe lesions may do better on spontaneous drawing tasks (where they have less dependence on reproducing a model figure) than on copying tasks (where they must accurately perceive and reproduce the figure). Patients with frontal lobe disorders have equal difficulty with drawing and copying, or they may exhibit environmental dependency and slavishly copy the presented figure while having greater difficulty with spontaneous drawing.

■ VISUOSPATIAL COGNITION AND MEMORY DISORDERS

In addition to the visual and visuospatial deficits described above, a variety of other cognitive and memory disturbances that primarily affect nonverbal visuospatial information processing have been described. Detection of most of these disturbances depends on use of structured neuropsychological tests, and most are more common after lesions of the right hemisphere than after lesions of the left hemisphere. Design fluency (Chapter 4, Figure 4–1) assesses the patient's ability to generate novel designs using four lines of equal length that touch at least one other line. The test is most difficult for patients with right-sided dorsolateral prefrontal lesions. The ability to synthesize fragments of objects into a whole and properly identify them is evaluated by tests such as the Hooper Visual Organization Test. In mental rotation tests, the patient is asked to imagine what a specific complex figure would look like if rotated and then must choose the answer from among several similar-appearing alternatives. Revisualization refers to the patient's ability to produce and describe an "internal" image of a named object (e.g., flag, bicycle, elephant). Patients with bilateral parietal lobe lesions may have deficits of internal revisualization and cannot imagine or describe a named object *(Charcot-Wilbrand syndrome)*.

Visual memory disturbances are best identified by showing patients figures that cannot be easily named (e.g., tangled lines) and asking them to draw the figures from memory or to choose the figures from a multiple-choice array after a delay. Right temporal lobe lesions have the greatest effect on visual memory. *Reduplicative paramnesia* is a syndrome in which the patients claim that they are simultaneously in two or more locations; it occurs in patients with lesions of both frontal lobes and the right temporal lobes (see Chapter 7).

TABLE 6–3. **Neuropsychiatric syndromes reported in patients with right-brain lesions**

Syndrome	Lesion location
Mania	Orbitofrontal cortex, caudate nucleus, thalamus, temporobasal region
Depression	Posterior hemispheric cortex
Anxiety	Temporal lobe (especially medially)
Delusions	Temporal lobe, temporoparietal region
Visual hallucinations	Geniculocalcarine radiations, occipital cortex, temporal lobe
Schizoid behavior	Posterior hemispheric cortex (especially if sustained early in life)
Hyposexuality	Temporal lobe
Receptive aprosodia	Temporal lobe
Executive aprosodia	Frontal lobe
Amusia	Temporal lobe
Visuospatial deficits	Parietal lobe
Dressing disturbance	Parietal lobe
Left spatial neglect	Parietal lobe
Anosognosia	Parietal lobe
Prosopagnosia	Medial occipitotemporal region
Facial discrimination defects	Parietal lobe
Environmental recognition defects	Medial occipitotemporal region
Voice recognition deficits	Parietal lobe
Voice discrimination deficits	Parietal lobe, temporal lobe
Nonverbal amnesia	Temporal lobe

■ NEUROPSYCHIATRIC SYNDROMES ASSOCIATED WITH RIGHT-BRAIN DYSFUNCTION

The disturbances addressed in this chapter are seen more commonly with right-hemisphere dysfunction than with left-brain disorders; therefore, they may coexist with neuropsychiatric syndromes that occur with right-brain lesions. The principal neuropsychiatric syndromes occurring in patients with right-brain dysfunction and their anatomical correlates are presented in Table 6–3. A contrasting set of syndromes occurring with left-brain lesions is provided in Table 6–4.

Mania occurs with lesions of the right hemisphere affecting the orbitofrontal, caudate, perithalamic, or temporobasal regions. Among patients with right-brain lesions, depression is most frequently associated with right posterior lesions and anxiety with

TABLE 6–4. **Neuropsychiatric syndromes associated with left-brain lesions**

Syndrome	Lesion location
Depression	Frontal lobe, temporal lobe, caudate nucleus
Depression with anxiety	Frontal cortex
Psychosis	Temporal lobe
Visual hallucinations	Geniculocalcarine radiations, occipital cortex, temporal lobe
Aphasia	Temporal lobe, inferior parietal region, frontal lobe (see Chapter 5)
Apraxia	Parietal lobe, frontal lobe, corpus callosum (see Chapter 5)
Primary acalculia	Parietal lobe (see Chapter 5)
Verbal amnesia	Temporal lobe (see Chapter 7)
Right spatial neglect	Parietal lobe
Denial of language deficit	Temporoparietal region

right temporal lobe dysfunction. Delusions occur with lesions of the right temporal lobe or temporoparietal junction regions. Misidentification syndromes such as the *Capgras syndrome* (the delusion that someone has been replaced by an identical-appearing impostor) are more common with right-sided lesions than with left-sided lesions. Patients with psychotic disorders accompanying right-brain lesions often have marked visual hallucinations with the delusions. Visual hallucinations without delusions may occur with lesions of the right hemisphere affecting the geniculocalcarine radiations, occipital cortex, or temporal lobes. Visual hallucinations are also common with lesions affecting the anterior visual structures (of either the right or left side) and compromising vision. Schizoid behavior has been reported among individuals who sustained right-brain lesions as children. Hyposexuality has been found to be more common after right-hemisphere lesions than after left-hemisphere lesions; hypersexuality may occur with manic syndromes associated with right-brain lesions.

■ REFERENCES AND RECOMMENDED READING

Aldrich MS, Alessi AG, Beck RW, et al: Cortical blindness: etiology, diagnosis, and prognosis. Ann Neurol 21:149–158, 1987

Bauer RM: Agnosia, in Clinical Neuropsychology, 3rd Edition. Edited by Heilman KM, Valenstein E. New York, Oxford University Press, 1993, pp 215–278

Benton A, Tranel D: Visuoperceptual, visuospatial, and visuoconstructive disorders, in Clinical Neuropsychology, 3rd Edition. Edited by Heilman KM, Valenstein E. New York, Oxford University Press, 1993, pp 165–213

Bogousslavsky J, Miklossy J, Regli F, et al: Subcortical neglect: neuropsychological, SPECT, and neuropathological correlations with anterior choroidal artery territory infarction. Ann Neurol 23:448–452, 1988

Carlesimo GA, Fadda L, Caltagirone C: Basic mechanisms of constructional apraxia in unilateral brain-damaged patients: role of visuoperceptual and executive disorders. J Clin Exp Neuropsychol 15:342–358, 1993

Cutting J: Study of anosognosia. J Neurol Neurosurg Psychiatry 41:548–555, 1978

Cutting J: The Right Cerebral Hemisphere and Psychiatric Disorders. New York, Oxford University Press, 1990

Damasio A, Yamada T, Damasio H, et al: Central achromatopsia: behavioral, anatomic, and physiologic aspects. Neurology 30:1064–1071, 1980

Damasio AR, Damasio H, Van Hoesen GW: Prosopagnosia: anatomic basis and behavioral mechanisms. Neurology 32:331–341, 1982

Heilman KM, Watson RT, Valenstein E: Neglect and related disorders, in Clinical Neuropsychology, 3rd Edition. Edited by Heilman KM, Valenstein E. New York, Oxford University Press, 1993, pp 279–336

Landis T, Cummings JL, Benson DF, et al: Loss of topographic familiarity: an environmental agnosia. Arch Neurol 43:132–136, 1986

Levine DN, Calvanio R, Rinn WE: The pathogenesis of anosognosia for hemiplegia. Neurology 41:1770–1781, 1991

Mendez MF: Visuoperceptual function in visual agnosia. Neurology 38:1754–1759, 1988

Mesulam M-M: A cortical network for directed attention and unilateral neglect. Ann Neurol 10:309–325, 1981

Rizzo M, Robin DA: Simultanagnosia: a defect of sustained attention yields insights on visual information processing. Neurology 40:447–455, 1990

Robinson RG, Starkstein SE: Current research in affective disorders following stroke. J Neuropsychiatry Clin Neurosci 2:1–14, 1990

Swindell CS, Holland AL, Fromm D, et al: Characteristics of recovery of drawing ability in left- and right-brain damaged patients. Brain Cogn 7:16–30, 1988

MEMORY AND ITS DISORDERS

Several memory systems have been defined. However, there are disagreements as to how to classify them, and differing terminologies have been proposed. A suggested scheme is outlined in Table 7–1. Most agree that there is a *short-term memory* (STM) store, a memory buffer, that holds information that is later to be discarded or stored. This is sometimes called *primary memory*. Some refer to *working memory*, STM with more than one capacity.

In contrast is *long-term memory* or *secondary memory*. Essentially, long-term memory is all that is not STM. There is good evidence that long-term memory is a separate system from STM. A classification system for long-term memory is shown in Figure 7–1.

Retrograde amnesia (RA) refers to the period of time for which memories are obliterated before an amnesia-producing event. *Posttraumatic amnesia* (PTA) is the length of time that memories are lost after a trauma, usually a cerebral injury. It is judged by the time it takes for a continuous stream of ongoing memory to return. Many patients report islands of memory after a head injury, which may reflect reality or may be a part of a posttraumatic confusional state. These are not included in the determination of the length of the PTA or the return of memory function. The amnesia due to sedative and anesthetic agents that a patient may receive in the course of early intensive treatment must always be considered a factor obscuring the PTA.

RA and PTA are both reflections of the severity of a cerebral injury. It is probably true that any trauma that leads to a clearly identifiable PTA will be associated with a loss of some cerebral neurons and that a PTA of 24 hours or longer represents a severe injury (see Chapter 13). An isolated PTA is frequent, but isolated RA virtually never occurs. Usually the PTA is longer than the RA, and a long RA in the presence of a short PTA is suggestive of a conversion disorder.

7

TABLE 7–1. **Memory systems**

System	Characteristics
Short term	Memory immediately after presentation without an intervening distracter
	Limited capacity
	Rapid decay
	Tested by digit span (capacity) or Brown-Peterson Task (duration)
Long term	Memory that is not short term
	Unlimited capacity; slow rate of forgetting
Declarative memory	Memory for facts (knowing that . . .)
	Accessible to consciousness (can be declared)
Semantic	Memory of general knowledge, world events (also called reference memory)
Episodic	Memory for ongoing autobiographical events (also called working memory)
Procedural memory	Memory for skills or modifiable cognitive operations (knowing how . . .)
	Spared in amnesia
	Includes classic conditioning
Implicit memory	A variety of procedural memory, demonstrated by completion of tasks that do not require conscious processing (e.g., completing word fragments)
Explicit memory	A variety of declarative memory
	Conscious recollection of recent events
Recall	
Retrieval	Activation of long-term memory traces
	Depends on frontal-subcortical circuits
Recognition	Ability to identify previously learned information
	Depends on initial information storage and the hippocampal-hypothalamic-thalamic system

Anterograde amnesia refers to impairment of retaining everyday information. It overlaps with the PTA if the patient is left with a severe memory disorder after cerebral injury. Persistent antero-

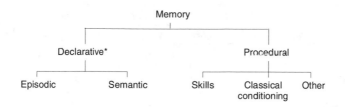

FIGURE 7–1. Classification of memory systems, excluding short-term memory. *Source.* Adapted from Squire 1987. *All tests described in Table 7–4 test this system.

grade amnesia is always associated with the presence of some RA and PTA.

Confabulation is often seen in patients with memory disorders. Completely erroneous answers are given to questions and elaborated on with apparent conviction. Confabulation is most commonly seen soon after the onset of a memory disorder.

■ ANATOMY OF MEMORY

By studying patients with various memory disorders and animal models, the underlying anatomy of memory has been defined. The crucial anatomical sites are shown in Table 7–2. The limbic system is central, but there are also extralimbic mechanisms. The latter relate to habit and skill learning, as procedural memory requires the function of the basal ganglia. STM depends on intact attentional mechanisms. The ability to repeat digits, a common test of STM, depends on intact linguistic processes.

The amygdala and the hippocampus, especially the CA_1 and CA_3 subfields, are involved in laying down memory traces and in anterograde amnesia. The hypothalamic and diencephalic structures most implicated are the mamillary bodies and the mediodorsal nucleus of the thalamus. The amygdala is involved in the

TABLE 7–2. **Some causes of the amnestic syndrome**

Etiology	Lesion site	Associated features
Stroke, posterior cerebral artery	Hippocampus	Homonymous hemianopia
Herpes simplex encephalitis	Hippocampus	Seizures, aphasia, Klüver-Bucy syndrome
Anoxia	Hippocampus	Anoxic episode
Hypoglycemia	Hippocampus	Diabetes and insulin
Head trauma	Hippocampus	History of trauma
Epilepsy surgery	Hippocampus	Bilateral disease
Tuberculous meningitis	Hippocampus	Tuberculoma; vascular occlusion
Alcoholism	Mamillary bodies or thalamus	Vitamin deficiency
Thiamine deficiency	Mamillary bodies or thalamus	Alcoholism or starvation
Neoplasms, especially around third ventricle	Thalamus	Headache, papilloedema

formation of long-term memory, notably in emotionally influenced memories, and in reinforcement.

The frontal lobes are also important in memory function. Patients with frontal lesions have impaired memory, especially for sequencing and ordering of events, as well as for retrieval of stored information. In some studies, retrograde memory impairment correlates with frontal impairments, and frontal lesions are often associated with confabulation. It has been suggested that patients with frontal lesions have a specific type of memory problem referred to as "forgetting to remember."

The main neurotransmitter identified with memory is acetylcholine. Cholinergic blockade in humans disrupts memory, whereas choline agonists may improve memory in some patients with dementia (see Chapter 9). The forebrain cholinergic system, ascending from the nucleus basalis of Meynert to the cortex and from the septal nuclei to the hippocampus, is crucial for memory function; patients with lesions at these sites have anterograde amnesias.

■ MEMORY DISORDERS IN CLINICAL PRACTICE

Memory is impaired secondarily in many states, for example, in anxiety and depression. Memory impairment is an integral aspect of conditions such as head injury and the dementias.

There are also primary memory disorders. *Amnesia* is an acquired disturbance of memory in which new information is not stored by any long-term memory system. There are several well-recognized etiologies (see Table 7–2). It is still unclear, from a psychological point of view, whether there is only one amnestic syndrome with several etiologies or several different syndromes.

The best-known amnestic syndrome is *Korsakoff's syndrome.* This syndrome is usually secondary to *Wernicke's encephalopathy,* which is itself due to thiamine deficiency. The latter presents with nystagmus, ophthalmoplegia, ataxia, peripheral neuropathy, and clouding of consciousness. After recovery from the acute state, the patient may be left with severe anterograde memory disturbance, confabulation, lack of insight, and a mood disturbance. These patients have intact STM: Korsakoff's syndrome is evident if there is a delay, or interference, between presentation of the stimuli and recording of a response.

Transient global amnesia is defined as a sudden global amnesia sometimes associated with minor clouding of consciousness that ends in recovery. It is more common in men in the 50- to 70-year age range. During the attack, personal identity is retained, significant persons are recognized, and motor skills are unimpaired. It lasts up to 24 hours, and when memory returns, there is an amnesia for the duration of the episode. There is an associated RA, which may be extensive but which quickly shrinks on recovery. Usually patients have only one attack, but multiple episodes are seen in some cases. The etiology of transient global amnesia is unclear, although epilepsy and transient ischemia have been implicated in some patients. Precipitating events can sometimes be identified, including stress, physical activity, and sexual intercourse. The electroencephalogram (EEG) is often abnormal during the attack.

Many neurologic disorders involve parts of the anatomical circuit for memory (Table 7–2). The dementias are described in Chapter 9, epilepsy in Chapter 8, and head trauma in Chapter 13. In all these conditions, the medial temporal areas often bear the brunt of the pathology, and complaints of disturbed memory are common.

Because the major blood supply of the hippocampus is the posterior cerebral artery, an occlusion of this vessel may lead to amnesia. This damage is often associated with a homonymous hemianopsia and sometimes with hemiplegia. In many cases, bilateral disease is present, but cases are described with unilateral infarction. Damage to the anterior cerebral artery and the anterior communicating artery leads to frontal lobe impairment, and it has been reported to lead to memory problems associated with confabulation. These problems probably result from damage to basal forebrain nuclei. Strokes of the thalamus may lead to amnesia; if bilateral, they may provoke a syndrome of amnesia and confusion. If the adjacent rostral brain stem is involved, there will be associated eye movement abnormalities.

Encephalitis sometimes selectively affects limbic structures. The main virus is herpes simplex type 1, which causes an acute necrotizing hemorrhagic encephalitis. The presentation is usually with focal neurologic signs and seizures, but the long-term sequelae are, in addition to seizures, usually behavioral. Amnesia is inevitable, and various manifestations of the Klüver-Bucy syndrome may be seen (see Chapter 8).

Memory impairment secondary to cerebral tumors is greatest when they involve subcortical structures, especially in and around the third ventricle, the thalamus, and the hippocampus.

Several neuropsychiatric treatments have been associated with transient amnesia. These include the benzodiazepines, electroconvulsive therapy (ECT), and anticholinergic drugs.

■ PSYCHOGENIC AMNESIAS

Psychogenic amnesia is currently classified as dissociative amnesia. Dissociative amnesia refers to an episode of "inability to recall important personal information, usually of a traumatic or stressful nature, that is too extensive to be explained by ordinary forgetfulness" (American Psychiatric Association 1994, p. 478). There is preservation of the ability to comprehend environmental information and to perform complex learned skills. It is a variety of dissociative disorder. Dissociation and repression are commonly held underlying mechanisms. It should be noted that psychogenic amnesia often occurs in the setting of a neurologic illness. A list of psychogenic amnesias, in approximate order of the length of the episode, is given in Table 7–3.

Situational amnesia may occur in isolation, in association with a psychologically significant or traumatic event, or as part of *posttraumatic stress disorder* (PTSD).

TABLE 7–3.   **Varieties of psychogenic amnesia**

Situational
Posttraumatic stress disorder[a]
Ganser's syndrome[b]
Psychogenic fugue
Hysterical dementia
Depressive dementia
Multiple personality disorder[b]
Histrionic personality disorder[a]

---

[a]Amnesia is commonly but not invariably present.
[b]The nosologic validity of these syndromes is least certain.

Fugues are episodes of wandering with amnesia. Patients remain in good contact with their surroundings, and when they emerge from the fugue, they may emerge with an amnesic gap, loss of their identity, and sometimes amnesia for their whole life.

The *Ganser syndrome* is a complex of hallucinations, cognitive disorientation, conversion disorder, and the symptom of approximate answers *(vorbeireden)*. It has been described in a number of settings and has been associated with head injury, depression, schizophrenia, epilepsy, chronic neurologic disorders, and malingering. Vorbeireden is the inability to answer simple questions correctly. Even though the nature of the questions is known, approximate answers are given. The absurd nature of these answers is striking.

Pseudodementia includes conditions such as the cognitive and memory impairments of depression (see Chapter 9), the Ganser syndrome, and hysterical dementia. Patients with hysterical dementia have a bizarre memory loss, associated with variable results on psychological testing and often associated with other conversion phenomena. This memory loss may be acute or chronic and may be precipitated by a head injury. Episodes of Ganser syndrome may be brief, whereas hysterical dementia may be chronic and relapsing.

■ DYSMNESIC STATES

In dysmnesic states, memory is not so much lost as it is distorted. These conditions are usually associated with a diagnosis of some underlying neurologic impairment or schizophrenia. The *delusional misidentification syndromes* include the *Capgras syndrome* and the *Fregoli syndrome*. In the former, the patient insists that a person, usually a close relative or friend, has been replaced by an impostor. In the Fregoli syndrome, the patient falsely identifies a familiar person, often a persecutor, in strangers. There is good evidence linking misidentification syndromes to the dysfunction of the right hemisphere and to frontal lobe disorders. *Déjà vu* and *jamais vu* are described in Chapter 1.

Reduplicative paramnesia is a related syndrome in which a patient is certain that a familiar place, person, object, or body part has been duplicated. It commonly presents when a patient insists that a familiar place (e.g., his or her hospital room) exists in an impossible location (e.g., his or her house).

TABLE 7–4.   **Some memory tests**

Digit span (auditory-verbal short-term memory)[**]
Corsi Blocks (visuospatial short-term memory)
General knowledge
Memory for word lists
Memory for stories
Memory for nonverbal material[**]
Rey-Osterrieth Complex Figure Test
  Recall of a figure
Recognition memory tasks—visual and verbal
  Patients are shown words,[*] faces,[*] objects, or shapes or are given word lists; after an interval, the same process is repeated with distracters, and those items already seen are to be identified
Hidden Objects Task
  Hide objects in view of patient
Brown-Peterson Task
  A test of the duration of short-term memory; patients are given items to remember, followed by a distraction task, and then a recall
Wechsler Memory Scale—Revised
  Twelve separate subtests, including above tests marked by double asterisk (**)
Photographs of famous faces
Photographs of famous landmarks
Word completion
Warrington Recognition Memory Test
  Includes above tests marked by single asterisk (*)

■ TESTS OF MEMORY FUNCTION

In practice, several tests are used in the clinic and in more formal neuropsychological settings. Some of the most common tests are listed in Table 7–4.

■ REFERENCES AND RECOMMENDED READING

American Psychiatric Association: Diagnostic and Statistical Manual of Mental Disorders, 4th Edition. Washington, DC, American Psychiatric Association, 1994

Benson DF, Marsden CD, Meadows JC: The amnestic syndrome of posterior cerebral artery occlusion. Acta Neurol Scand 50:133–145, 1974

Damasio AR, Graff-Radford NR, Eslinger PJ, et al: Multimodal amnesic syndrome following bilateral temporal and forebrain damage. Arch Neurol 42:252–259, 1985

Damasio AR, Graff-Radford NR, Eslinger PJ, et al: Amnesia following basal forebrain lesions. Arch Neurol 42:263–271, 1985

Kopelman M: Memory and the temporal lobes, in The Temporal Lobes and the Limbic System. Edited by Trimble MR, Bolwig T. Petersfield, England, Wrightson Biomedical, 1992, pp 199–210

Lewis S: Brain imaging in a case of the Capgras syndrome. Br J Psychiatry 150:117–121, 1987

Mace CJ, Trimble MR: Psychogenic amnesia, in Memory Disorders: Research and Clinical Practice. Edited by Yanagihara T, Petersen RC. New York, Marcel Dekker, 1991, pp 429–457

Squire LR: Memory and the Brain. New York, Oxford University Press, 1987

Stuss DT, Alexander MP, Liberman A, et al: An extraordinary form of confabulation. Neurology 28:116–172, 1978

Warrington EK: Recognition Memory Test. Windsor, England, NFER-Nelson, 1984

Yanagihara T, Petersen RC: Memory Disorders: Research and Clinical Practice. New York, Marcel Dekker, 1991

Yudofsky SC, Hales RE (section eds): The neuropsychiatry of memory, in American Psychiatric Press Review of Psychiatry, Vol 12. Edited by Oldham JM, Riba MB, Tasman A. Washington, DC, American Psychiatric Press, 1993, pp 661–833

EPILEPSY AND LIMBIC SYSTEM DISORDERS

A number of conditions have a predilection to affect the limbic areas of the brain and consequently lead to behavior disorders. Included is one form of epilepsy, temporal lobe epilepsy (TLE), in which the seizure focus is in the medial limbic portions of that lobe. In this chapter, epilepsy is first discussed with special reference to TLE.

■ EPILEPSY

Epilepsy is a cerebral disorder in which the patient has a liability to recurrent seizures. Seizures are the main symptom of epilepsy. Although 1 person in 20 has a seizure in his or her lifetime, the prevalence of epilepsy is about 0.5%.

The currently used classification of epilepsy is shown in Table 8–1. Table 8–2 shows the classification of seizures.

Partial seizures are those in which clinical and electroencephalographic (EEG) changes suggest a focal onset. Further classification depends on whether consciousness is impaired during the attack. *Generalized seizures* are those in which the first clinical and EEG changes suggest bilateral abnormalities with widespread disturbance in both hemispheres. *Absence seizures* are usually associated with regular 3-Hz-per-second spike and slow-wave activity on EEG. *Tonic-clonic seizures* are classic grand mal episodes; *myoclonic seizures* are sudden, brief, jerklike contractions that may be focal or generalized. *Cursive seizures* refer to running during attacks, and *gelastic seizures* refer to laughing.

Automatisms refer to automatic motor acts carried out in a state of altered consciousness during or after seizures, for which there is usually amnesia. They generally last less than 15 minutes. Persistent focal seizures are referred to as *epilepsia partialis continua*. *Rasmussen's syndrome* refers to a viral encephalitis that

8

TABLE 8–1. **Classification of the epilepsies**

---

1. Localization-related (focal, local, partial) epilepsies and syndromes
    Idiopathic
    Symptomatic
2. Generalized epilepsies or syndromes
    Idiopathic
    Idiopathic or symptomatic (e.g., West's syndrome)
    Symptomatic
3. Undetermined as to whether they are generalized or focal
4. Special syndromes (e.g., febrile convulsions)

Source. Adapted from International League Against Epilepsy 1985.

presents as persistent focal seizures, with slowly progressive neurologic deterioration. There is evidence of brain atrophy, usually unilateral.

In *status epilepticus,* recurrent seizures occur without return of consciousness between attacks. In nonconvulsive status epilepticus, patients present with prolonged episodes of abnormal behavior due to continuous seizures of either the complex partial or absence type. Schizophrenia-like states, associated with variable degrees of confusion (which sometimes may be only slight), may be seen.

The classification of the epilepsies is essentially one of syndromes, not diseases. *West's syndrome* consists of infantile spasms

---

TABLE 8–2. **Classification of seizures**

---

1. Partial (focal, local) seizures
    Simple partial (retention of consciousness)
    Complex partial (may begin with simple partial)
    Partial seizures evolving to secondarily generalized seizures
2. Generalized seizures
3. Unclassified seizures

Source. Adapted from International League Against Epilepsy 1981.

in association with a specific EEG pattern called hypsarrhythmia. Hypsarrhythmia is characterized by high-amplitude slow waves at frequencies of 1–7 Hz, mixed with sharp waves and spikes of varying amplitude, morphology, duration, and site. Onset is in the first year of life. The *Lennox-Gastaut syndrome* occurs in children up to about 8 years of age and presents with multiple seizure types, a markedly disturbed EEG, and mental handicap. In the *reflex epilepsies* seizures are provoked by cognitive, emotional, sensory, or motor events.

The principal causes of epilepsy are shown in Table 8–3. *Kindling* is a phenomenon in which repeated subthreshold electrical stimulations lead to the subsequent development of seizures and a permanent increase in the epileptogenicity of the brain

TABLE 8–3. **Principal causes of seizures**

Metabolic	**Traumatic**
Hypoglycemia	Head injuries
Hypomagnesemia	**Infections**
Fluid and electrolyte disturbances	Viral encephalitis
Acute intermittent porphyria	Acquired immunodeficiency syndrome
Amino acid disorders	Cytomegalovirus
Neurologic	Toxoplasmosis
Tumors	Meningitis
Cerebrovascular accident	Cysticercosis
Degenerative and storage disorders	Syphilis
Demyelinating diseases (uncommon)	**Drug withdrawal**
	Alcohol
Sturge-Weber syndrome	Benzodiazepines
Tuberous sclerosis	Barbiturates
Poisons	**Vitamin deficiency**
Lead	Pyridoxine
Strychnine	**Temperature**
	Fever

kindled. As such, it is an experimental model of seizure development and not a clinical phenomenon.

■ PSYCHIATRIC DISORDERS OF EPILEPSY

A classification of behavioral disorders encountered in patients with epilepsy is shown in Table 8–4. The distinction between *ictal* and *interictal* syndromes is not always clear. In some patients, prolonged postictal psychotic states occur, merging into interictal psychoses in the setting of clear consciousness. Furthermore, *forced normalization* is a seizure-related state that seems interictal (see below).

There are few epidemiologic studies of the incidence and prevalence of interictal psychopathology. Estimates are that around 20%–30% of epileptic patients demonstrate psychopathology at some time, mainly anxiety and depression. The lifetime prevalence for an episode of psychosis is in the region of 4%–10%, increasing to 10%–20% in patients with TLE.

The *interictal personality syndrome* is characterized by the features shown in Table 8–5. Aggression is not a specific compo-

---

TABLE 8–4. **Classification of psychiatric disorders of epilepsy**

Seizure related

    Peri-ictal (including auras and prodromes)

    Parictal (associated with increased seizures and clusters)

    Forced normalization (associated with sudden cessation of seizures)

    Postictal (associated with a disorganized electroencephalogram and clouding of consciousness following a seizure)

Interictal

    Schizophrenia-like psychoses

    Paranoid states

    Affective disorders

    Anxiety states

    Personality disorders

---

nent. High-risk factors for the latter include diffuse neurologic illness, low socioeconomic class, and a dysfunctional family.

The *episodic dyscontrol syndrome* refers to sudden episodes of spontaneously released violence, often with minimal provocation, that are brief and terminate abruptly. They may be precipitated by small amounts of alcohol, and patients later show remorse. Evidence of subtle cerebral damage may be present, including an abnormal EEG with slow rhythms (theta) over the temporal lobes and neuroimaging evidence of medial temporal lobe pathology. The condition may be associated with epilepsy but is clearly distinct from it. The term *epileptic equivalent* is a bad one; a patient either has epilepsy or does not.

Depression is the most common interictal syndrome. However, many patients present with a chronic dysphoria with high anxiety levels and irritability rather than a typical major affective disorder. Suicide is higher in epileptic than in nonepileptic populations, especially in patients with TLE. The following have been associated with depression in epilepsy: barbiturates and drugs acting at the γ-aminobutyric acid (GABA)–benzodiazepine receptor complex, low serum and red cell folate levels, late-onset epilepsy, and a decrease in the frequency of seizures.

The psychoses typically have a paranoid or schizophrenia-like presentation. The latter often include Schneiderian first-rank symptoms (Chapter 3, Table 3–3) in the absence of personality deterioration, affective warmth being maintained. This presentation is most often seen with TLE, especially with left-sided or

TABLE 8–5. **Features of the interictal personality syndrome**

Hyperreligiosity, philosophical and mystical preoccupation

Disordered sexual function

Hypergraphia (tendency for excessive and compulsive writing)

Irritability

Viscosity (stickiness of thought—bradyphrenia)

bilateral seizure foci. Risk factors for the development of psychoses are shown in Table 8–6.

Many patients with TLE can be shown to have a specific pathology: *mesial temporal sclerosis* (MTS). This condition is often unilateral, and there is loss of neurons with gliosis in the hippocampus and related structures. The CA_1 region is especially vulnerable. There is an association between MTS and prolonged febrile convulsions of childhood. Hamartomas and tumors also occur. Hamartomas arise from disordered cell differentiation and migration during development and resemble tumors but are not neoplastic. A common site of pathology is in medial temporal structures. Schizophrenia is associated with lesions at the same sites. It is therefore of substantial interest that the development of a schizophrenia-like psychosis is associated with TLE. A difference between idiopathic schizophrenia and the schizophrenia-like states of epilepsy is that the pathology of schizophrenia does not seem to include gliosis. The similarities are 1) the disorganization of neurons; 2) the involvement primarily of the hippocampus; 3) the fact that in both syndromes the pathology is established in

---

TABLE 8–6. **Risk factors for the development of psychoses in epilepsy**

Age at onset: around puberty

Interval: period between onset of seizures and onset of psychosis is around 14 years

Sex: bias to females

Seizure type: complex partial; automatisms

Seizure frequency: may be diminished; forced normalization in a subgroup

Epilepsy syndrome: localization related, symptomatic

Seizure focus: temporal, especially left sided or bilateral

Neurology: left-handed; abnormal neurologic examination

Pathology: gangliogliomas and hamartomas

Electroencephalogram: mediobasal focus

very early life, whereas the main manifestations appear years later, particularly in late adolescence and early adulthood; and 4) the fact that both syndromes present with a wide range of psychological and behavioral symptoms and signs.

Forced normalization refers to the observation that certain patients develop psychiatric symptoms when their seizures come under control. Originally, forced normalization was thought to involve only psychoses, but other behaviors are now recognized in this setting, including depression, anxiety, agitation, and conversion disorders. In children, attention-deficit/hyperactivity disorder or conduct disturbance can result. The EEG "normalizes" during the behavior disturbances, and as the disturbances resolve, the EEG becomes abnormal again.

The phenomenon is usually of acute onset, but in some patients, an interictal psychosis gradually emerges over time as seizure frequency declines. It is usually precipitated by anticonvulsant drugs, especially benzodiazepines, barbiturates, ethosuximide, lamotrigine, and vigabatrin. The clinical counterpart, when EEG evidence is unavailable, is called *alternative psychosis*.

■ PSEUDOSEIZURES

The term *pseudoseizures* is problematic. Patients have seizures, but they do not have epilepsy. Nonepileptic seizures, nonepileptic attack disorder, or pseudoepileptic seizures better describe the problem.

In some cases, the clinical pattern so resembles epilepsy that videotelemetry is essential before a diagnosis can be made. After generalized tonic-clonic seizures, prolactin levels reliably rise dramatically (to over 1000 IU/L) from a normal baseline, but they fail to do so after a pseudoseizure. This test is less reliable for complex partial seizures and not reliable for simple partial seizures and status epilepticus. Blood must be sampled within 20 minutes of an attack.

Patients with *frontal lobe epilepsies* (FLEs) may present with sudden-onset, short-duration seizures that look bizarre, with much

TABLE 8–7. **Nonpsychiatric differential diagnosis of pseudoseizures**

Hypoglycemia
Syncope and vasovagal attacks
Migraine, especially basilar migraine
Vertebrobasilar ischemia
Transient ischemic attacks
Transient global amnesia
Sleep disorders
  Parasomnias
    Rapid eye movement (REM) related
      REM behavior disorder
      Nightmares
    Non-REM related
      Night terrors
      Somnambulism
  Hypersomnias
    Narcolepsy
    Cataplexy

motor movement that is often wild and with little or no postictal mental confusion. The EEG may be remarkably normal. These seizures are badly termed *pseudo-pseudoseizures*.

The nonpsychiatric and psychiatric differential diagnoses of pseudoseizures are given in Tables 8–7 and 8–8.

TABLE 8–8. **Psychiatric disorders associated with pseudoseizures**

Panic attacks	Déjà vu experience
Depersonalization and derealization	Depressive fugues
	Rage attacks
Paroxysmal anxiety	Catatonic behaviors

■ OTHER TEMPORAL LOBE DISORDERS

Although TLE is the most common temporal lobe syndrome seen in neuropsychiatry, other pathologies also have a predilection for damaging the limbic system. Head injury is discussed in Chapter 13. Three viruses that often affect this region of the brain are those causing *rabies, encephalitis lethargica,* and *herpes encephalitis.* The latter is caused by herpes simplex virus type 1 (HSV-1) and has a high mortality rate; survivors often display psychopathology. Part or all of the *Klüver-Bucy syndrome* (see Table 8–9) may be present. In addition, there is often severe amnesia, irritability, distractibility, and dysphoria with apathy.

Cerebral tumors include gliomas and hamartomas. The latter occur anywhere in the brain but seem to be more associated with psychopathology, especially psychosis, when they occur in the temporolimbic areas.

Limbic encephalitis has been associated with systemic carcinoma.

Some patients have temporal lobectomies for relief of intractable TLE. The indications for the operation are given in Table 8–10. A number of patients develop postoperative psychiatric syndromes, including transient or more severe affective disorder, anxiety states, and psychoses. Suicide is one cause of postoperative death.

Pharmacotherapies for psychiatric syndromes associated with epilepsy are discussed in Chapter 14.

TABLE 8–9. **Main components of the Klüver-Bucy syndrome**

Hypermetamorphosis (overattention to external stimuli)	Agnosia
	Inappropriate sexual activity
Tendency to explore objects orally	Tameness, loss of fear

TABLE 8–10.	**Indications for temporal lobectomy**

Intractable seizures

Failure to respond to all available medications

Evidence for a unilateral focus, preferably by magnetic resonance imaging or positron-emission tomography, sometimes by electroencephalogram or other indices alone

Evidence that memory function can be sustained by the remaining temporal lobe (usually tested by the amobarbital sodium [Wada or Amytal] test)

Patient wants to have the operation

■ REFERENCES AND RECOMMENDED READING

Bear D: Behavioural changes in TLE: conflict, confusion, challenge, in Aspects of Epilepsy and Psychiatry. Edited by Trimble MR, Bolwig T. Chichester, England, Wiley, 1986, pp 19–30

Corsellis JAN, Goldberg GJ, Norton AR: Limbic encephalitis, and its association with carcinoma. Brain 91:481–496, 1968

Davison K, Bagley CR: Schizophrenia-like psychoses associated with organic disorders of the CNS, in Current Problems in Neuropsychiatry. Edited by Herrington RN. Kent, England, Headley Brothers, 1969, pp 113–184

Fenwick P: Precipitation and Inhibition of seizures, in Epilepsy and Psychiatry. Edited by Reynolds EH, Trimble MR. Edinburgh, Scotland, Churchill Livingstone, 1981, pp 242–263

Fenwick P: Aggression and epilepsy, in Aspects of Epilepsy and Psychiatry. Edited by Trimble MR, Bolwig T. Chichester, England, Wiley, 1986, pp 31–60

Glaser G, Pincus JH: Limbic encephalitis. J Nerv Ment Dis 149:59–68, 1969

Heath RG: Common characteristics of epilepsy and schizophrenia. Am J Psychiatry 118:1013–1026, 1962

International League Against Epilepsy: Proposal for a revised clinical and electroencephalographic classification of epileptic seizures. Epilepsia 22:489–501, 1981

International League Against Epilepsy: Proposal for a classification of the epilepsies and epileptic syndromes. Epilepsia 26:268–278, 1985

Monroe R: Episodic Behavior Disorders. Boston, MA, Harvard University Press, 1970

Perez MM, Trimble MR: Epileptic psychosis—diagnostic comparison with process schizophrenia. Br J Psychiatry 137:245–249, 1984

Robertson MM, Trimble MR: Depressive illness in patients with epilepsy: a review. Epilepsia 24 (suppl 2):S109–S116, 1983

Scheibel A: Are complex partial seizures a sequela of temporal lobe dysgenesis? in Neurobehavioral Problems in Epilepsy. Edited by Smith DB, Treiman DM, Trimble MR. New York, Raven Press, 1991, pp 59–78

Slater E, Beard AW: The schizophrenia-like psychoses of epilepsy. Br J Psychiatry 109:95–150, 1963

Taylor DC: Factors influencing the occurrence of schizophrenia-like psychoses in patients with epilepsy. Psychol Med 5:249–254, 1975

Trimble MR: The Psychoses of Epilepsy. New York, Raven, 1991

Waxman SG, Geschwind N: The interictal behavior syndrome of TLE. Arch Gen Psychiatry 32:1580–1586, 1975

Wolf P, Trimble MR: Biological antagonism and epileptic psychosis. Br J Psychiatry 146:272–276, 1985

DEMENTIA AND DELIRIUM

Disorders of intellectual function may involve disruption of a single neuropsychological domain such as memory (the amnesias) or language (the aphasias), or they may affect multiple cognitive functions. The two syndromes characterized by multiple simultaneous intellectual deficits are delirium and dementia. This chapter addresses the clinical features and causes of these two syndromes. Clinical criteria developed to identify the different dementias are emphasized.

■ DELIRIUM

Attentional disturbance is the single most salient feature of delirium. Delirium is manifested by an inability to sustain, direct, or appropriately shift attentional resources. Sustained concentration and freedom from distraction are compromised, as manifested by fluctuating arousal and erratic attentional shifts, particularly in response to environmental events. Patients may exhibit a wide spectrum of arousal: they may not be fully aroused and may lapse easily into sleep, or they may be hyperaroused with exaggerated vigilance and prominent startle reactions.

Abnormalities of attention result in impaired performance of most other cognitive activities. The presence of an attentional disturbance can usually be demonstrated by the digit span test (asking the patient to repeat a series of digits read aloud by the examiner) or by a continuous performance test (such as asking the patient to raise his or her hand each time the examiner reads the letter *A* in a series of letters read aloud at a rate of 1 per second over a 30-second period). The coherence of thought processes is affected, leading to incoherent speech output and rapid shifting from one topic to another.

Anomia and nonaphasic misnaming (systematic misnaming, often reflecting the person's past experience, such as when a

9

delirious mechanic calls a thermometer a hammer and a stethoscope a wrench) are linguistic changes that may accompany delirium. Agraphia may be particularly prominent in deliria; patients make errors of omission and repetition when writing words, phrases, and sentences. A variety of memory abnormalities may occur. The patient may be so inattentive that information is not registered, and both recall and recognition are disturbed; or registration may occur but recall is unpredictable, with the patient exhibiting impaired recall with preserved recognition memory. Constructional abilities are abnormal and are characterized by poor organization and omission of details. Neuropsychological abilities such as calculation and executive functions (described in Chapter 4) are highly vulnerable to attentional disturbances and are error ridden in delirious patients. Visual hallucinations and persecutory delusions are common in delirious episodes.

Abnormalities of the neurologic examination are evident in many delirious patents. An action tremor is often present, and myoclonic jerks are common. Asterixis—the sudden interruption of muscle tone resulting in an abrupt disruption of sustained muscle activity (such as the "liver flap" demonstrable in the outstretched hands of patients with hepatic encephalopathy)—is present in many types of deliria. A slurred dysarthria may be evident.

Toxic and metabolic disturbances are by far the most common cause of deliria (Table 9–1). In rare instances, delirium is produced by focal brain lesions, typically located in the posterior temporal–inferior parietal region of the right hemisphere. Bilateral occipital lesions may also produce a delirious state. Patients with dementia commonly become delirious with minor infections, fever, and electrolyte disturbances. Dementia cannot be diagnosed until the delirium resolves.

Laboratory abnormalities reflect the underlying etiology of the delirium. Serum or urine drug assays, blood gases, and serum chemistry tests are commonly used to diagnose intoxications, hypoxic states, and electrolyte or glucose disturbances responsible for

---

TABLE 9–1.   **Causes of delirium**

Cardiopulmonary disease
Congestive heart failure
Pneumonia
Chronic obstructive pulmonary disease
Asthma with respiratory compromise
Gastrointestinal disturbances
Hepatic encephalopathy
Pancreatitis
Genitourinary abnormalities
Renal failure
Urinary tract infection
Intoxications
Alcohol
Illicit drugs
Over-the-counter agents (e.g., sleeping aids)
Prescribed medications
Neurologic disorders
Meningitis
Encephalitis
Right temporal–parietal lesions
Bilateral occipital lesions

---

delirium. Diagnosis of more unusual causes of delirium requires specialized testing. The electroencephalogram (EEG) is nearly always abnormal in patients with toxic and metabolic disorders and may help distinguish delirium from other neuropsychiatric disorders. The EEG is typically normal in patients with depression, schizophrenia, and early degenerative dementias, whereas marked generalized slowing is characteristic of toxic-metabolic encephalopathies.

Features most useful in distinguishing delirium and dementia are summarized in Table 9–2. Each dementia and each cause of delirium has unique features. Table 9–2 contrasts the features common to most dementias with those of typical deliria.

TABLE 9–2. **Contrasting features of dementia and delirium**

Feature	Delirium	Dementia
Onset	Acute or subacute	Insidious
Course	Fluctuating	Persistent
Duration	Limited	Chronic
Attention	Impaired	Intact until advanced stages
Language	Incoherent	More coherent
Speech	Slurred dysarthria	Dysarthria uncommon
Visual hallucinations	Common	Uncommon
Tremor	Common	Uncommon
Myoclonus	Common	Occurs in only a few types of dementia
Electroencephalogram	Prominent abnormalities	Mild changes

■ DEMENTIA

Dementia is a clinical syndrome characterized by an acquired persistent impairment in at least three of the following domains of function: language, memory, visuospatial skills, executive abilities, and emotion. Dementia is a syndrome that can be produced by a wide variety of disorders; it may be reversible or irreversible. It is distinguished from mental retardation by its acquired nature and by the requirement that the patient's function has declined from a previously more competent level. It is distinguished from delirium primarily by its persistent course and the other features noted in Table 9–2. It is differentiated from amnesia or aphasia by the multiplicity of behavioral deficits. Dementia may be of mild, moderate, or marked severity. It is conventional to limit the use of the term to syndromes of sufficient severity to interfere with the patient's occupational performance or social interactions. In most cases, dementia is progressive (e.g., Alzheimer's disease), but patients with trauma, postinfectious states, and some stroke syndromes may exhibit a stable course, or there may be partial remission of cognitive deficits.

Two general types of dementia have been recognized within the generic dementia syndrome: cortical dementia and subcortical dementia. The distinguishing features of these two syndromes are presented in Table 9–3. The etiologies of dementia and their approximate frequencies in a clinic population are shown in Table 9–4.

TABLE 9–3. **Distinguishing characteristics of cortical and subcortical dementias**

Function	Cortical dementia	Subcortical dementia
Psychomotor speed	Normal	Slowed
Language	Involved	Spared
Memory		
Recall	Impaired	Impaired
Recognition	Impaired	Spared
Remote	Temporal gradient present	Temporal gradient absent
Executive function	Less involved	More involved
Depression	Less common	More common
Apathy	Less common	More common
Motor system	Spared until late	Involved early
Anatomy	Cerebral cortex	Subcortical structures and dorsolateral prefrontal cortex projecting to head of caudate nucleus
Examples	Alzheimer's disease	Huntington's disease, HIV encephalopathy, lacunar state

Note. HIV = human immunodeficiency virus.

TABLE 9–4. **Etiologies of dementia**

Dementia	Frequency (%)
Alzheimer's disease	50–60
Vascular dementia	10–30
Depression	5–15
Alcohol-related dementia	1–10
Metabolic disturbances	1–10
Toxic disturbances	1–10
Hydrocephalus	1–5
Anoxia brain injury	1–2
Central nervous system infections	1–2
Brain tumors	1–2
Brain trauma	1–2
Subdural hematoma	1–2
Other	10–20

Note. The reported frequencies are drawn from reports of populations seeking care in outpatient clinics and do not reflect the distribution of dementing diseases among inpatients or in epidemiologic surveys.

ALZHEIMER'S DISEASE

Alzheimer's disease (AD) is a progressive neurodegenerative disorder that produces a clinical syndrome termed *dementia of the Alzheimer type* (DAT). AD has an insidious onset and progresses gradually to death. The disorder is age related and becomes increasingly common after age 65 years. Survival is typically about 10 years from the time of diagnosis. The earliest changes usually include impaired memory and a change in personality characterized by indifference. Examination at this stage will typically reveal subtle alterations in language and visuospatial abilities. As the disease progresses, memory changes become more pronounced and include both learning of new information and remote recall. The visuospatial disability worsens; the patients become disoriented easily and cannot copy or draw accurately.

Language abnormalities begin with anomia and then progress to a transcortical type of aphasia with fluent verbal output, impaired comprehension of spoken speech, and relatively preserved repetition (Chapter 5). Abstraction, calculation, and executive functions are also compromised in this stage of the illness. Motor, somatosensory, and visual function remain intact. In the final phases of the disease, essentially no memory function can be demonstrated, and language is reduced to echolalia, palilalia, and incoherent verbalization. The patient loses the ability to walk, and incontinence occurs. Delusions, anxiety, and dysphoria are common in AD, and agitation is a frequent behavioral disturbance of more advanced patients. In unusual cases, the disease may begin with delusions, aphasia, apraxia, or marked visuospatial disturbances.

Table 9–5 lists the criteria used to make a clinical diagnosis of AD. Definite, probable, and possible AD are recognized. A diagnosis of *definite AD* is made when the patient meets all clinical criteria for probable AD and then has biopsy or autopsy findings compatible with the diagnosis (described below). *Probable AD* is the diagnosis given to patients who manifest clinical findings indicative of AD; who have had other illnesses excluded by clinical assessment, laboratory studies, and neuroimaging; and who have not had a biopsy. The diagnostic accuracy rate of these criteria when applied strictly is approximately 85%. *Possible AD* is the diagnosis used when patients exhibit atypical clinical features (e.g., progressive impairment of memory but sparing of other neuropsychological abilities) or have another illness that can cause dementia but is thought not to be responsible for the patient's cognitive deficits (e.g., hypothyroidism or vitamin B_{12} deficiency that has been treated).

There is no diagnostic test for AD. Serum, urine, and routine cerebrospinal fluid (CSF) tests are normal. EEG will usually reveal slowing of the dominant posterior rhythm and an increasing abundance of theta- and delta-range slowing as the disease progresses. P300 evoked responses are delayed after clinical symptoms have appeared. Structural imaging such as computed tomography (CT)

TABLE 9–5. **Diagnostic criteria for definite, probable, and possible Alzheimer's disease**

Definite AD

Clinical criteria for probable AD

Histopathologic evidence of AD (autopsy or biopsy)

Probable AD

Onset between ages 40 and 90 years

No disturbance of consciousness (e.g., not in a delirium)

Dementia established by clinical examination and documented by mental status questionnaire

Dementia confirmed by neuropsychological testing

Progressive worsening of memory and other cognitive functions

Deficits in memory and in at least one other cognitive function (language, visuospatial abilities, calculation, executive function, praxis, gnosis)

Absence of systemic disorders or other brain diseases capable of producing a dementia syndrome (diseases such as Parkinson's disease and frontal lobe degenerations are identified and excluded by clinical examination; other potential causes of dementia are detected and excluded by laboratory tests and neuroimaging)

Possible AD

Presence of a systemic disorder or other brain disease capable of producing dementia but not thought to be the cause of the patient's dementia

Gradually progressive decline in a single intellectual function in the absence of any other identifiable cause (e.g., memory loss, aphasia)

Unlikely AD

Sudden onset

Focal neurologic signs

Seizures or gait disturbance early in the course of the illness

---

Note. AD = Alzheimer's disease.

---

and magnetic resonance imaging (MRI) reveals nonspecific cerebral atrophy. Single photon emission computed tomography (SPECT) typically demonstrates diminished cerebral blood flow; the most marked reductions are in the inferior parietal and parietotemporal junction areas. Positron-emission tomography

(PET) shows diminished neuronal metabolism in AD, and the regions with the most severe changes are in the inferior parietal and parietotemporal junction areas. The regional alterations demonstrated by SPECT and PET reflect the anatomic pattern of neuropathologic changes in AD and provide characteristic findings supportive of the clinical diagnosis.

At autopsy, the brain is atrophic with enlarged sulci and dilated ventricles. Histologic changes include neuron loss, astrocytic gliosis, neuritic plaques, neurofibrillary tangles, and amyloid angiopathy. These changes are most abundant in the medial temporal lobes, temporal poles, and posterior temporal–inferior parietal regions. The frontal lobes are moderately affected; primary motor and sensory cortex and subcortical structures are spared or are much less involved.

The pathogenesis of AD remains to be elucidated. Two basic processes have emerged as particularly important in the cascade of events leading to cell death. First, abnormalities of the amyloid precursor protein (APP) or of the metabolism to amyloid lead the accumulation of β-amyloid in neuritic plaques and leptomeningeal blood vessels. Amyloid may be toxic to neurons and contributes to cell death. Second, there is abnormal phosphorylation of the tau protein associated with neuron microtubules, leading to formation of neurofibrillary tangles. Inheritance of mutations of chromosomes 21 and 14 appears to cause the abnormalities of amyloid processing, whereas inheritance of the ApoE-4 allele of chromosome 19 may facilitate both accumulation of amyloid and formation of neurofibrillary tangles.

Behavioral disturbances in patients with AD are managed with conventional psychotropic agents (see below and Chapter 14); side effects are common and dosages should be minimized. In addition, pharmacotherapy of cognitive deficits is available and helps some AD patients. Tacrine, a cholinesterase inhibitor, produces improvement in cognition in 30%–50% of patients who are able to tolerate the higher doses (120–160 mg daily in four divided doses) of the drug. An average response is improvement, to the level of performance present 6–12 months earlier in the illness. Occasional patients exhibit marked improvement. Tacrine does not alter the underlying disease process and deterioration eventually occurs. Tacrine is potentially hepatotoxic, and weekly monitoring of serum alanine aminotransferase (ALT) levels is required for 6 weeks after each increase in dosage and every 3 months during stable dosing periods. Administration begins with 10 mg four times daily and increases every 6 weeks by 40 mg per day (10 mg qid, 20 mg qid, 30 mg qid, 40 mg qid).

VASCULAR DEMENTIA

Vascular dementia (VAD) is the second most common cause of dementia in elderly persons, accounting for between 10% and 30% of patients. The diagnostic criteria for VAD are presented in Table 9–6. The critical features include the presence of dementia, evidence of cerebrovascular disease, and a compelling association between these two characteristics.

VAD may be produced by several types of cerebrovascular pathology, and several VAD syndromes are recognized. Multiple cerebral emboli produce multifocal infarction, usually involving the cerebral cortex. Sustained hypertension leads to fibrinoid necrosis of arterioles with lacunar infarction of the basal ganglia, thalamus, and deep hemispheric white matter (lacunar state) and ischemic demyelination of the periventricular regions and deep white matter (Binswanger's disease). Combinations of deep and superficial infarctions may also occur.

Cortical infarctions produce deficits in cortically mediated functions (resulting in aphasia, amnesia, agnosia, and apraxia), and subcortical infarctions produce the syndrome of subcortical dementia (see Table 9–3). Parkinsonism with mixed pyramidal and extrapyramidal dysfunction commonly accompanies the subcortical form of VAD. Strategic infarctions are small, critically located lesions that disrupt multiple cognitive functions. The angular gyrus syndrome is the most common example of a strategic-

---

TABLE 9–6. **Diagnostic criteria for vascular dementia (VAD)**

Definite VAD

Clinical criteria for probable VAD

Autopsy demonstration of appropriate ischemic brain injury with no other cause found for the dementia

Probable VAD

Dementia

Decline from a previously higher level of cognitive functioning

Impairment of two or more cognitive domains

Deficits severe enough to interfere with activities of daily living and not due to physical effects of stroke alone

Not in a delirium

Psychosis, aphasia, or sensorimotor impairment not so severe as to preclude neuropsychological testing

No other disorder capable of producing a dementia syndrome is present

Cerebrovascular disease

Focal neurologic signs consistent with stroke

Neuroimaging evidence of appropriate (extensive or strategic) vascular lesions

A relationship between the dementia and the cerebrovascular disease as evidenced by

Onset of dementia within 3 months of a recognized stroke, or

Abrupt deterioration, fluctuating course, or stepwise progression of the cognitive deficit

Possible VAD

Dementia with focal neurologic signs but without neuroimaging confirmation of definite cerebrovascular disease

Dementia with focal neurologic signs but without a clear temporal relationship between dementia and stroke

Dementia and focal neurologic signs but with a subtle onset and variable course of cognitive deficits

---

infarct dementia; the syndrome is comprised of alexia, agraphia, anomia, acalculia, right-left confusion, finger agnosia, ideomotor apraxia, and verbal memory impairment in association with lesions of the left angular gyrus (Chapter 5). Neuropsychiatric disturbances are common in VAD. Depression and psychosis are evident in nearly half of all patients. Apathy and irritability also frequently occur.

DEMENTIA OF DEPRESSION

The dementia of depression—also known as "depressive pseudodementia"—occurs primarily in elderly individuals and is characterized by slowness of thought, poor memory, and impaired executive function. Aphasia is not present. Depression with sadness, feelings of helplessness and worthlessness, sleep disturbance, and appetite changes is usually evident, and anxiety and delusions frequently accompany the cognitive changes. Agitation or retardation may be the predominant motor manifestation. The diagnosis is confirmed by recovery of cognitive function with successful treatment of the mood disorder. Psychopharmacologic treatment or electroconvulsive therapy may produce recovery of mood and cognition. CT shows more marked atrophy in patients with the dementia of depression than in depressed patients of similar age without intellectual impairment. The prognosis of the dementia of depression is controversial. Some follow-up studies have shown that the syndrome is the harbinger of a degenerative dementia, whereas others suggest that recurrent depressive episodes are common, but permanent dementia does not supervene.

FRONTAL LOBE DEGENERATIONS

Frontotemporal dementias (FTDs) are idiopathic neurodegenerative diseases that produce lobar atrophy of the frontal and/or temporal lobes. Asymmetric degeneration is common, with predominant right- or left-sided changes. Three principal types of FTDs are recognized: 1) Pick's disease, characterized by neurons containing Pick bodies and ballooned Pick cells; 2) frontal lobe degeneration (FLD) without distinctive histologic features evidencing neuron loss and gliosis without definitive Pick bodies or

Pick cells; and 3) dementia in conjunction with motor neuron disease (frontal lobe degeneration–amyotrophic lateral sclerosis [FLD-ALS] complex).

Clinically, FTD usually begins between 50 and 70 years of age. It is inherited as an autosomal-dominant disorder in a minority of patients. FTD has an insidious onset with prominent changes in personality or language. Behavior alterations in FTD include disinhibition, impulsiveness, tactlessness, and impaired social judgment. In some patients, apathy predominates. The language disturbance of FTD typically begins with an anomia and proceeds to a reserved verbal output with mutism or marked speech stereotypies (saying the same thing repeatedly). Repetition may be preserved longer than other types of verbal output. Memory, copying, and calculations are largely spared until the middle stages of the illness, and assessing these abilities aids in distinguishing FTD from AD. Depression, obsessive-compulsive behavior, and psychosis are common in FTD. Parkinsonism may occur in the later stages of the illness, and fasciculations (contractions of motor unit visible as episodic dimpling of muscles or vermiform movements of the tongue) are present in patients with the FLD-ALS complex.

HYDROCEPHALUS

Hydrocephalus may be nonobstructive (hydrocephalus ex vacuo produced by tissue loss) or obstructive. The latter may be noncommunicating (produced by obstruction of CSF flow within the ventricular system or between the ventricular system and the subarachnoid space via the outflow foramina of the fourth ventricle) or communicating (normal-pressure hydrocephalus [NPH]). The obstruction to CSF flow in NPH is usually in the arachnoid granulations of the superior sagittal sinus, preventing absorption of CSF into the venous system.

Noncommunicating hydrocephalus is more common in children and presents with increased intracranial pressure, headache, papilledema, and sixth-nerve palsy. The most common causes are congenital malformations of the midbrain aqueduct, intracranial tumors, and acute meningitis. NPH presents with dementia, incontinence, and gait abnormalities (ataxia, apraxia, or parkinsonism). It usually follows cerebral trauma, meningitis, or encephalitis but may have no identifiable antecedents. NPH is diagnosed by identifying hydrocephalus on CT or MRI and showing abnormal CSF flow characteristics on radionuclide cisternography. Diversion of CSF to the intraperitoneal space via a lumboperitoneal or ventriculoperitoneal shunt is the necessary intervention.

CENTRAL NERVOUS SYSTEM INFECTIONS WITH DEMENTIA

Dementia can be produced by chronic meningitis, slow viruses, and prions (proteinaceous infectious particles), or it may occur as a static state after encephalitis (particularly herpes encephalitis) (Table 9–7).

Human immunodeficiency virus (HIV) encephalopathy may be the presenting manifestation of acquired immunodeficiency syndrome (AIDS) or may evolve after the infection has affected other organ systems. The disease is produced by a retrovirus; the principal risk factors for infection are unprotected sex with an infected homosexual partner and intravenous drug administration with contaminated needles. The cognitive changes have the features of subcortical dementia (Table 9–3), with prominent apathy. Rigidity, ataxia, tremor, seizures, and myoclonus may accompany the dementia syndrome. Positive HIV serology in the absence of evidence of other causes of mental status changes (particularly opportunistic central nervous system [CNS] infections) support the diagnosis. At autopsy, inflammatory changes and multinucleated giant cells are identified in the cerebral white matter. Treatment with azidothymidine (AZT) may improve intellectual function or retard the progress of the disorder; psychostimulants or antidepressants may improve arousal and mood.

TABLE 9–7. **Principal infectious causes of dementia**

Chronic meningitis
  Fungal
    Cryptococcus
    Histoplasmosis
  Parasitic
    Cysticercosis
    Toxoplasmosis
  Bacterial
    Tuberculosis
    Syphilis
    Lyme disease
Slow viruses
  Human immunodeficiency virus encephalopathy
  Subacute sclerosing panencephalitis (SSPE)
  Progressive multifocal leukoencephalopathy (PML)
Prions
  Creutzfeldt-Jakob disease
  Gerstmann-Straüssler-Scheinker disease
Postencephalitic states
  Herpes encephalitis

Creutzfeldt-Jakob disease is a rapidly progressive prion disorder that produces dementia, extrapyramidal dysfunction, pyramidal tract signs, and myoclonus. Prions are infectious proteinaceous particles also known as unconventional viruses. Patients with Creutzfeldt-Jakob disease usually succumb within 6–12 months of onset. The EEG has characteristic periodic discharges in most patients, although they may not appear until late in the course. No treatment is available. Pathologically, the principal changes include marked astrocytic hypertrophy and spongiform changes of the cortex.

MISCELLANEOUS DEMENTIA SYNDROMES

Alcohol, solvent inhalation (glue sniffing), industrial or occupational solvent exposure, polydrug abuse, and chronic excessive use of over-the-counter drugs are toxic conditions that produce cognitive impairment. Medications administered for control of behavioral disturbances or systemic illness may cause or exacerbate intellectual abnormalities. Medical disorders including cardiopulmonary diseases, anemia, gastrointestinal conditions and deficiency states, and endocrinopathies may produce dementia syndromes. Dementia is present in many patients with movement disorders (Chapter 10), vascular and collagen-vascular diseases (Chapter 11), brain tumors (Chapter 11), multiple sclerosis and other diseases of the white matter (Chapter 12), and cerebral trauma (Chapter 13).

Lewy bodies (extranuclear intracytoplasmic bodies composed of a neurofilamentous core and surrounding halo) are present in several types of dementia including Parkinson's disease with dementia and a rare disorder called cortical Lewy body disease. In addition, they are found in the cerebral cortex of a substantial number of patients with late-onset degenerative dementia. These patients also have cortical neuritic plaques but few neurofibrillary tangles; it is currently unresolved whether this is a separate type of dementia (senile dementia of the Lewy body type) or a variant of AD (Lewy body variant of AD).

DEMENTIA IN CHILDREN

Children may exhibit static encephalopathies manifested by mental retardation and delayed acquisition of developmental milestones, or they may have dementia syndromes characterized by loss of previously acquired skills. Progressive dementia is rare in children and requires thorough assessment. Table 9–8 lists the principal causes of dementia in infants, children, and adolescents and the laboratory tests most helpful in their identification. Inherited white

TABLE 9–8. **Causes of dementia in infants, children, and adolescents and the laboratory tests most helpful in establishing a diagnosis**

Brain disorder	Laboratory tests
Inherited white matter disorders	
Alexander's disease	CT, MRI (frontal lobe demyelination)
Cerebrotendinous xanthomatosis	Serum cholestanol
Polycystic lipomembranous osteodysplasia	CT, hand films, skin biopsy
Adrenoleukodystrophy	Serum very long chain fatty acids
Metachromatic leukodystrophy	Leukocyte arylsulfatase A
Krabbe's disease (globoid cell leukodystrophy)	Leukocyte galactocerebroside β-galactosidase
Inherited gray matter disorders	
Lafora's disease	Liver or skeletal muscle biopsy
Ceroid lipofuscinosis	Urinary dolichols, brain biopsy
G_{M1} gangliosidosis	Leukocyte G_{M1} β-galactosidase
G_{M2} gangliosidosis	Leukocyte hexosaminidase A
Gaucher's disease	Leukocyte β-glucocerebrosidase
Niemann-Pick disease	Liver biopsy, leukocyte sphingomyelinase
Mucopolysaccharidosis	Leukocyte α-N-acetylglucosaminidase
Wilson's disease	Serum copper and ceruloplasmin
Fabry's disease	Leukocyte α galactosidase
Miscellaneous disorders	
Mitochondrial encephalopathies	Serum lactate/pyruvate levels
HIV encephalopathy	Serum HIV antibodies
Leigh's disease	CT, MRI (bilaterally symmetric lesions of basal ganglia)
Neuroacanthocytosis	CT, nerve-conduction studies, acanthocytes
Pseudoxanthoma elasticum	Skin biopsy
Schizophrenia (dementia praecox)	Clinical assessment

Note. CT = computed tomography. HIV = human immunodeficiency virus. MRI = magnetic resonance imaging.

matter diseases with children, many of which begin in childhood, are discussed in Chapter 12.

■ ASSESSMENT OF DEMENTIA

A careful history and thorough mental status examination (Chapters 1 and 3–7) provide the information critical for identification and differential diagnosis of dementia and delirium. The initial assessment provides clues to the diagnosis and generates hypotheses that will be confirmed or disconfirmed by laboratory tests and neuroimaging. Accurate diagnosis is necessary for treatment and for counseling the patient and patient's family regarding prognosis, hereditary risks, and management. Table 9–9 outlines the standard evaluation of the demented patient; additional tests are chosen based on specific historic, occupational, clinical, neuroimaging, and preliminary laboratory information.

■ TREATMENT OF DEMENTIA

Behavior disorders associated with dementia and delirium are treated with psychotropic agents based on the patient's predominant symptoms. Psychosis usually responds to low doses of neuroleptic agents, and agitation is treated with neuroleptics, trazodone, buspirone, carbamazepine, or propranolol. Tricyclic agents with few anticholinergic side effects, selective serotonin reuptake inhibitors (fluoxetine or others), and other antidepressants with favorable side effect profiles are used in dementia with depression or the dementia of depression. Anxiety in depression usually resolves with benzodiazepines, buspirone, or propranolol. Benzodiazepines that are well metabolized by elderly patients include oxazepam, lorazepam, and temazepam. Insomnia may respond to treatment with trazodone, a benzodiazepine (e.g., temazepam), or a sedating neuroleptic. These agents are discussed in Chapter 14, and management of specific conditions associated with dementia is de-

TABLE 9–9. **Standard assessment of the dementia patient**

Laboratory tests

  Complete blood count

  Erythrocyte sedimentation rate

  Electrolytes, blood glucose, blood urea nitrogen (BUN)

  Serum calcium and phosphorus

  Thyroid-stimulating hormone (TSH)

  Serum vitamin B_{12} level

  Fluorescent treponemal antibody absorption test (FTA-ABS)

Neuroimaging

  Computed tomography or magnetic resonance imaging

Useful systemic assessments

  Electrocardiogram

  Chest X ray

  Urinalysis

Optional tests

  Lumbar puncture

  EEG and quantitative EEG

  Single photon emission computed tomography

  Positron-emission tomography

  Serum antiphospholipid antibodies

  Serum or urine drug tests

  Radionuclide cisternography

  Serum human immunodeficiency virus antibodies

Note. EEG = electroencephalogram.

scribed in Chapters 10–13. The use of tacrine in AD is described above.

Appropriate use of psychotropic agents in dementia can delay nursing home placement and diminish the use of restraints with patients residing in institutions. Patients may also improve with nonpharmacologic environmental manipulations, and these should be tried before initiating pharmacotherapy. The principals of avoiding any unnecessary drugs, minimizing polypharmacy, beginning with low drug dosages, increasing dosages slowly, and constantly monitoring for side effects are particularly applicable to patients with dementia.

Caring for patients with dementia is stressful, and assessment of the caregiver is an essential element of dementia treatment.

■ REFERENCES AND RECOMMENDED READING

Albert MS, Levkoff SE, Reilly C, et al: The Delirium Symptom Interview: an interview for the detection of delirium symptoms in hospitalized patients. J Geriatr Psychiatry Neurol 5:14–21, 1992

American Psychiatric Association: Diagnostic and Statistical Manual of Mental Disorders, 4th Edition. Washington, DC, American Psychiatric Association, 1994

Coker SB: The diagnosis of childhood neurodegenerative disorders presenting as dementia in adults. Neurology 41:794–798, 1991

Cummings JL, Benson DF: Dementia of the Alzheimer type: an inventory of diagnostic clinical features. J Am Geriatr Soc 34:12–19, 1986

Cummings JL, Benson DF: Dementia: A Clinical Approach, 2nd Edition. Boston, MA, Butterworth-Heinemann, 1992

Cummings JL, Miller B, Hill MA, et al: Neuropsychiatric aspects of multi-infarct dementia and dementia of the Alzheimer type. Arch Neurol 44:389–393, 1987

Devinsky O, Bear D, Volpe BT: Confusional states following posterior cerebral artery infarction. Arch Neurol 45:160–163, 1988

Eagger SH, Levy R, Sahakian BJ: Tacrine in Alzheimer's disease. Lancet 337:989–992, 1991

Francis J, Martin D, Kapoor WN: A prospective study of delirium in hospitalized elderly. JAMA 263:1097–1101, 1990

Ishii N, Nishahara Y, Imamura T: Why do frontal lobe symptoms predominate in vascular dementia with lacunes? Neurology 36:340–345, 1986

Jagust WJ, Budinger TF, Reed BR: The diagnosis of dementia with single photon emission computed tomography. Arch Neurol 44:258–262, 1987

Jagust WJ, Friedland RP, Budinger TF, et al: Longitudinal studies of regional cerebral metabolism in Alzheimer's disease. Neurology 38:909–912, 1988

Jorm AF, Korten AE, Henderson AS: The prevalence of dementia: a quantitative integration of the literature. Acta Psychiatr Scand 76:465–479, 1987

La Rue A, Spar J, Hill CD: Cognitive impairment in late-life depression: clinical correlates and treatment implications. J Affect Disord 11:179–184, 1986

Lipowski ZJ: Delirium: Acute Confusional States. New York, Oxford University Press, 1990

Lund and Manchester Groups: Clinical and neuropathological criteria for frontotemporal dementia. J Neurol Neurosurg Psychiatry 57:416–418, 1994

McKhann G, Drachman D, Folstein M, et al: Clinical diagnosis of Alzheimer's disease: report of the NINCDS-ADRDA Work Group, Department of Health and Human Services Task Force on Alzheimer's Disease. Neurology 34:939–944, 1984

Miller BL, Cummings JL, Villaneuva-Meyer J, et al: Frontal lobe degeneration: clinical, neuropsychological, and SPECT characteristics. Neurology 41:1374–1382, 1991

Mori E, Yamadori A: Acute confusional state and acute agitated delirium. Arch Neurol 44:1139–1143, 1987

Navia BA, Jordan BD, Price RW: The AIDS dementia complex, I: clinical features. Ann Neurol 19:517–524, 1986

Osborn AG: Diagnostic Neuroradiology. St. Louis, MO, Mosby, 1994

Overman W Jr, Stoudemire A: Guidelines for legal and financial counseling of Alzheimer's disease patients and their families. Am J Psychiatry 145:1495–1500, 1988

Quality Standards Subcommittee of the American Academy of Neurology: Practice parameters for diagnosis and evaluation of dementia. Neurology 44:2203–2206, 1994

Reichman WE, Cummings JL: Diagnosis of rare dementia syndromes: an algorithmic approach. J Geriatr Psychiatry Neurol 3:73–83, 1990

Roman GC: Senile dementia of the Binswanger type. JAMA 258:1782–1788, 1987

Roman GC, Tatemichi TK, Erkinjuntti T, et al: Vascular dementia: diagnostic criteria for research studies. Report of the NINDS-AIREN International Work Group. Neurology 43:250–260, 1993

Swearer JM, Drachman DA, O'Donnell BF, et al: Troublesome and disruptive behaviors in dementia. J Am Geriatr Soc 36:784–790, 1988

MOVEMENT DISORDERS 10

Movement disorders are produced by dysfunction of the basal ganglia, and these deep gray matter structures are increasingly recognized to be critically important in cognition and emotion as well as in motor function. There are three important corollaries with respect to the role of the basal ganglia in mental function: 1) basal ganglia disorders are frequently accompanied by abnormalities of intellectual integrity, mood, motivation, and personality; 2) many psychotropic agents affect the basal ganglia and produce movement disorders as side effects; and 3) many idiopathic psychiatric disorders have motoric manifestations.

This chapter describes the neuropsychiatric disturbances that accompany movement disorders. Parkinson's disease (PD) and parkinsonism are discussed first, followed by the hyperkinetic movement disorders and tremors.

■ PARKINSON'S DISEASE

DEMOGRAPHY

PD is an idiopathic degenerative disease that affects selected nuclei of the brain stem (substantia nigra, ventral tegmental area, locus coeruleus) and produces depletion of neurotransmitters (dopamine, norepinephrine) from neurochemical systems originating in these nuclei. PD has a prevalence in the general population of 100–200/100,000. The mean age at onset of PD is between 58 and 62 years, and the duration of illness averages 13–14 years. Men are slightly more likely to have PD than women; the disorder has little genetic risk.

CLINICAL FEATURES

The cardinal motor features of PD are bradykinesia, rigidity, and rest tremor. Bradykinesia is manifested by hesitation before initiating movements, slowness in executing movements, and a paucity of spontaneous movement and gesture. Reduced arm swing when walking and a tendency to take several small steps when turning are additional evidence of bradykinesia. Hypophonia of speech, an expressionless ("masked") face, and micrographia when writing are also manifestations of bradykinesia. Two types of rigidity occur in PD. Most patients have a plastic type of rigidity with increased resistance to passive flexion and extension of the limbs. In addition, if tremor is present, a cogwheel type of ratchet resistance can be detected while assessing tone. The typical rest tremor of PD is a large-amplitude, 4–6 cycles per second (cps), alternating flexion-extension movement that usually involves the fingers and wrist but may involve other body parts (lips, tongue, legs). Rest tremor is most apparent when the patient is in a state of alert repose; it disappears with action of the involved limb and is absent in sleep. Tremor is exaggerated by stress. An action tremor (small amplitude, 10–12 cps) that appears with motion and disappears with rest occurs in some patients with PD.

In PD, results of structural neuroimaging such as computed tomography (CT) and magnetic resonance imaging (MRI) are normal or show mild to moderate cerebral atrophy. Glucose metabolism demonstrated by positron-emission tomography (PET) and cerebral perfusion imaged by single photon emission computed tomography (SPECT) are usually normal. PET fluorodopa scans reveal diminished transmitter uptake into the basal ganglia.

PATHOLOGY

The substantia nigra, ventral tegmental area, and locus coeruleus are routinely affected in PD. There is depigmentation and Lewy body formation in the substantia nigra and locus coeruleus and loss of neurons from the involved structures. The nucleus basalis of Meynert, a basal forebrain nucleus, is involved in some but not all patients, and some patients have Alzheimer-type pathology of the cerebral cortex. Lewy bodies are common in a restricted distribution in the cerebral cortex of patients with PD, and a few patients have widespread cortical Lewy bodies.

Several types of neurochemical changes are present in PD. Dopamine is synthesized in the substantia nigra and transported to putamen, caudate, and medial temporal and medial frontal lobe regions. In PD, dopamine depletion is most marked in the putamen. Norepinephrine is synthesized in the locus coeruleus, and the pathologic changes in this region in PD are associated with variable cortical noradrenergic deficits. Serotonin is reduced in the striatum, substantia nigra, and hippocampus in PD. Acetylcholine is synthesized by choline acetyltransferase, which is manufactured by neurons in the nucleus basalis. Cholinergic function is reduced in PD patients who have atrophy of nucleus basalis.

TREATMENT

PD responds to treatment with dopaminergic agents, and failure of a patient to improve with therapy challenges the accuracy of the diagnosis. Two approaches to treatment are currently pursued: 1) treatment that slows the progress of the disease and delays or prevents cell death, and 2) treatment that provides relief of symptoms but has no effect on the underlying disease process. Selegiline is a monoamine oxidase B (MAO-B) inhibitor that inhibits the formation of hydroxy radicals generated in the course of the catabolism of dopamine and exogenous toxins suspected to play a role in the pathogenesis of PD. These hydroxyl molecules damage cell members and lead to cell death; thus, MAO-B inhibition reduces oxidative damage, preserves cell membranes, and enhances cell survival (see also the discussion of selegiline in Chapter 14). Unanimity on whether this is selegiline's principal mode of action has not been achieved.

Symptomatic relief in PD can be provided by anticholinergic agents, dopamine precursors (levodopa, usually administered in a fixed combination with carbidopa [Sinemet], to prevent peripheral metabolism of the levodopa), facilitation of dopamine release and inhibition of reuptake (amantadine), and dopamine receptor agonists (bromocriptine, pergolide). Table 10–1 lists drugs used in the treatment of PD, their dosages, and their principal side effects.

TABLE 10–1. **Agents used in the treatment of Parkinson's disease**

Class and agent	Usual dosage	Side effects of the class
Monoamine oxidase B inhibitor		
Selegiline	5 mg po in A.M.; 5 mg at noon	Insomnia, hallucinations, delusions
Anticholinergics		
Benztropine	2–6 mg/day	Urinary retention, constipation, blurred vision, confusion
Trihexyphenidyl	4–8 mg/day	
Dopamine release facilitation		
Amantadine	200–300 mg/day	Hallucinations, delusions
Dopamine precursor		
Levodopa	300–2000 mg/day	Hallucinations, delusions, euphoria, mania, hypersexuality, confusion
Sinemet[a]	10/100 tid to 25/250 qid	
Dopamine receptor agonist		
Bromocriptine	6–30 mg/day	Hallucinations, delusions, euphoria, mania, hypersexuality, confusion
Pergolide	1–5 mg/day	

[a]Sinemet is a fixed combination of levodopa and carbidopa; the latter is a dopamine β-hydroxylase inhibitor that prevents the peripheral metabolism of levodopa.

DEMENTIA AND COGNITIVE ALTERATIONS

Intellectual impairment is common in PD. Approximately 40% of PD patients meet criteria for overt dementia as detected by routine mental status examination, and an additional 30% have more subtle cognitive impairments. Many of the patients with mild cognitive decline exhibit the characteristics of subcortical dementia (Chapter 9). The causes of intellectual deterioration in PD are multiple. Severe dopamine deficiency can produce the syndrome of subcortical dementia. Patients with pathologic changes in the nucleus basalis and the brain stem dopaminergic nuclei have combined cholinergic and dopaminergic deficits and are reported to have more severe dementia than those with changes limited to the dopaminergic nuclei. Patients with widespread cortical Lewy bodies also show dementia, and patients with Alzheimer-type cortical pathology have the clinical features of both PD and Alzheimer's disease.

DEPRESSION

Dysphoric mood is frequent in PD, occurring in half of the patients. The depressive syndrome has atypical features: sadness and feelings of hopelessness and helplessness are common, but guilt and self-deprecation are rare. Anxiety is common in conjunction with depression, and suicide and delusional depression are infrequent. Depressed patients tend to have lower levels of 5-hydroxyindoleacetic acid, the principal metabolite of serotonin, in their cerebrospinal fluid. PET reveals that glucose metabolism of the frontal lobes is decreased in depressed compared with nondepressed PD patients. The depression does not correlate with the severity of the motor deficit and must be treated separately with antidepressant agents or electroconvulsive therapy (Chapter 14).

OTHER NEUROPSYCHIATRIC DISORDERS

Anxiety is common in both depressed and nondepressed PD patients. Apathy is the most common personality alteration of PD and has been identified in both depressed and nondepressed patients. Psychosis is uncommon in PD except after treatment with dopaminergic or anticholinergic agents.

DRUG-INDUCED NEUROPSYCHIATRIC DISORDERS

Dopamine is one of the most powerful psychoactive agents in clinical use. It functions in a variety of nervous system circuits that mediate motor, cognitive, and emotional activities. When administered to PD patients, it has the ability to produce a remarkable resurrection of motor abilities, but it can also produce a panoply of motoric and behavioral side effects. Chorea, tics, and myoclonus are motor expressions of dopamine excess in PD. Hallucinations occur in 30%, delusions in 10%, anxiety in 10%, euphoria in 10%, and hypersexuality in 1% of PD patients treated with dopaminergic agents. These complications usually occur in the absence of delirium, although high doses of dopaminergic agents can produce an acute confusional state. Most of these manifestations are best managed by reducing the dose of the dopaminergic drug. Dopaminergic psychosis can be managed by administering low doses of a neuroleptic agent such as thioridazine or use of atypical antipsychotic agents such as clozapine or risperidone. PD patients are unusually sensitive to the sedating effects of clozapine, and doses in the range of 25–100 mg be adequate to control the psychosis without producing intolerable side effects. Risperidone is also sedating, and doses of 0.5–3 mg are usually sufficient to control drug-related psychosis. When behavioral changes are induced by anticholinergic agents, the patient is usually in a delirium with marked attentional deficits, fluctuating arousal, and reduced coherence of thought.

■ PARKINSONISM

Parkinsonian syndromes are clinical conditions that resemble PD but lack the cardinal features or deviate from the classic disorder in some other important way. Parkinsonian patients typically manifest bradykinesia and rigidity but often lack tremor. Non-PD parkinsonian syndromes also tend to respond poorly to treatment with dopaminergic therapy. The most common non-PD parkinsonian syndromes are described briefly, and a more extensive differential diagnosis is provided in Table 10–2.

PROGRESSIVE SUPRANUCLEAR PALSY

Progressive supranuclear palsy (PSP) is manifested by a characteristic tetrad: supranuclear gaze palsy, axial rigidity, pseudobulbar palsy, and dementia. Supranuclear gaze palsy is evidenced by the loss of vertical gaze (down gaze is compromised before up gaze, and volitional saccadic eye movements are impaired before pursuit movements); axial rigidity refers to increased tone in truncal and neck muscles imparting an extended posture to the patient; pseudobulbar palsy in PSP features a marked dysarthria. The dementia of PSP has subcortical features (Chapter 9). Depression and obsessive-compulsive disorder (OCD) have been described in PSP patients. Treatment is with antiparkinsonian agents (described above), but the response is modest at best. At autopsy, patients have cell loss, neurofibrillary tangles, and granulovacuolar degeneration involving the neurons of the midbrain, globus pallidus, and thalamus. Neuroimaging (CT or MRI) may reveal brain stem atrophy, and SPECT or PET usually demonstrate diminished perfusion or metabolism of the frontal lobes.

VASCULAR PARKINSONISM

Vascular parkinsonism occurs in patients with multiple small vessel occlusions producing infarctions in the basal ganglia and the deep hemispheric white matter. The most common causes of the small vessel disease are sustained hypertension (leading to lipohyalinosis of arterioles) and diabetes. Patients typically exhibit subcortical dementia, parkinsonism with gait changes and bradykinesia but little tremor, and pyramidal tract signs (spasticity, exaggerated muscle stretch reflexes, pseudobulbar palsy, and Babinski signs). Occasional patients may improve with antiparkinsonian agents. Depression, psychosis, apathy, and irritability

TABLE 10–2. **Differential diagnosis of parkinsonism**

Parkinsonian disorder	Key clinical features
Parkinson's disease	Bradykinesia, rigidity, rest tremor, treatment responsive
Postencephalitic parkinsonism	Followed encephalitis lethargica epidemic (1918–1926); occasional current cases, oculogyric crises, asymmetric motor changes, prominent neuropsychiatric alterations
Progressive supranuclear palsy	Axial rigidity, vertical gaze paralysis, pseudobulbar palsy
Rigid Huntington's disease	Early onset, family history, minor choreiform movements
Shy-Drager syndrome	Prominent impotence, postural hypotension, incontinence
Striatonigral degeneration	Similar to Parkinson's disease but unresponsive to treatment
Olivopontocerebellar atrophy	Cerebellar and pyramidal system abnormalities
Cortical-basal degeneration	Asymmetric onset, marked apraxia, and visuospatial deficits
Cortical Lewy body disease	Dementia similar to Alzheimer's disease with visual hallucinations and fluctuations in disability
Rett's syndrome	Autism, ataxia, stereotyped hand movements in girls
Wilson's disease	Kayser-Fleischer corneal rings, low serum ceruloplasmin
Idiopathic basal ganglia calcification	Calcified basal ganglia on CT, normal serum calcium
Hallervorden-Spatz disease	Globus pallidus mineralization on CT and MRI
Vascular parkinsonism	Spastic rigidity, asymmetric reflexes, Babinski signs
Dementia pugilistica	Extensive history of boxing
Hydrocephalus	Markedly enlarged ventricles on CT or MRI

(continued)

TABLE 10–2.	Differential diagnosis of parkinsonism *(continued)*
Creutzfeldt-Jakob disease	Rapid progression, pyramidal signs, periodic EEG pattern
Syphilis	Positive serum FTA-ABS and CSF VDRL
Drug-induced parkinsonism	Neuroleptic treatment, tremor absent or minimal
Carbon monoxide	Carbon monoxide exposure, globus pallidus lesions on CT
Hypoparathyroidism	Calcified basal ganglia on CT, reduced serum calcium

Note. CSF = cerebrospinal fluid. CT = computed tomography. EEG = electroencephalogram. FTA-ABS = fluorescent treponemal antibody absorption. MRI = magnetic resonance imaging. VDRL = Venereal Disease Research Laboratory.

are the most common neuropsychiatric features of vascular parkinsonism. The terms *lacunar state* and *Binswanger's disease* are used when infarctions predominate in the basal ganglia and white matter, respectively.

DRUG-INDUCED PARKINSONISM

Parkinsonism may be induced by dopamine-blocking agents including neuroleptics (phenothiazines, butyrophenones) and agents used to control gastrointestinal disorders (compazine, metoclopramide). Patients typically manifest bradykinesia and rigidity and are less likely to exhibit tremor. Older patients are more susceptible to this side effect than younger patients. Amelioration of the syndrome is usually accomplished by reducing the dosage of the inciting agent and temporarily treating the patient with anticholinergic agents or amantadine. Levodopa and dopamine receptor agonists are used in the treatment of drug-induced parkinsonism only if the motor symptoms are extreme. These agents may exacerbate a psychotic disorder.

■ HUNTINGTON'S DISEASE

CLINICAL FEATURES

Huntington's disease (HD) is an autosomal-dominant neurodegenerative disease associated with a mutation on chromosome 4. The disease commonly begins between the ages of 35 and 40 years, and the duration is 12–16 years. Late-onset (after age 50 years) and juvenile-onset (under age 20 years) cases occur. The disease is equally common in men and women; inheritance from the father is more likely among early-onset cases.

HD is a hyperkinetic disorder with choreic movements affecting the proximal and distal limbs, trunk, face, and speech musculature. Gait abnormalities and dysarthria are prominent. A supranuclear gaze palsy occurs in a majority of patients. A rigid variant with parkinsonism is much less common and is most frequent in the juvenile form of the disease. Structural imaging (CT, MRI) typically reveals atrophy of the caudate nuclei in HD, and PET demonstrates reduced metabolism in these nuclei.

Neuroleptic medications suppress the chorea. There is no intervention available that retards the course of the disease or improves the accompanying dementia.

PATHOLOGY

At autopsy, there is marked cell loss in the caudate nuclei and the putamina, moderate loss of cells from thalamic nuclei, and variable neuron dropout in the cerebral cortex. Medium-sized spiny neurons are disproportionately affected in the striatum. γ-Aminobutyric acid (GABA) is depleted in the affected regions in HD. Concentrations of substance P, cholecystokinin, and metenkephalin are also severely reduced.

NEUROPSYCHIATRIC MANIFESTATIONS

A variety of neuropsychiatric disorders occur in HD. All of the patients manifest subcortical dementia (Chapter 9), and the cognitive alterations are the earliest manifestations in some cases. Personality changes are ubiquitous throughout the illness and include irritability, disinhibition, and conduct disorders. Patients may have personality alterations closely resembling intermittent explosive disorder or antisocial personality disorder. Depression occurs in 40%–50% of patients, and mania is present in approximately 2%. Suicide is a major complication of the depressive disorder. Psychosis is present in 5%–15% of patients. OCD has been observed in some cases. Behavioral alterations precede the onset of the chorea in approximately one-third of cases. Treatment of the behavioral disorders of HD involves the use of conventional psychotropic agents (Chapter 14). Carbamazepine is usually superior to lithium for the management of mania in HD.

■ NON-HUNTINGTON'S DISEASE CHOREAS

Chorea occurs in a wide array of neurologic and systemic disorders. Two common causes of chorea are described below, and the extended differential diagnosis is presented in Table 10–3.

TARDIVE DYSKINESIA

Tardive dyskinesia (TD) is a choreiform disorder that occurs after chronic administration of dopamine-blocking agents. Diagnosis of TD requires that the patient have a cumulative exposure of at least 3 months to a neuroleptic or other dopamine-blocking agent and that other causes of chorea be excluded. The movements of TD are typically small-amplitude choreic jerks involving the tongue, lips, and fingers. Truncal dyskinesia and foot and toe movements are also common. The chorea is present at rest and increased by distraction; it is reduced by action of the affected limb, directing attention to the movements, and asking the patient to volitionally suppress the movements. There is little subjective awareness of TD. Once it occurs, TD is stable in a majority of patients, although a small number progress to severe chorea and disability. Resolution

TABLE 10–3. **Differential diagnosis of chorea**

Choreic disorder	Key clinical features
Huntington's disease	Autosomal dominant, dementia, atrophy of caudate on CT or MRI
Benign familial chorea	Early onset, nonprogressive, no dementia
Neuroacanthocytosis	Chorea and tics, peripheral neuropathy, acanthocytes
Chorea with stroke	Acute onset, hemiballismus early
Cerebral palsy	Anoxic early-life episode
Kernicterus	Elevated bilirubin in infancy
Sydenham's chorea	Follows streptococcal A infection, positive anti-DNase B titer
Chorea gravidarum	Pregnancy, history of Sydenham's chorea
Chorea with SLE	Positive ANA and anti-double-stranded DNA
Antiphospholipid antibody syndrome	Positive lupus anticoagulant and anticardiolipin A and B antibodies
Acquired hepatocerebral degeneration	Liver failure
Polycythemia vera	Elevated hematocrit
Hyperthyroidism	Low TSH, elevated T_4
Tardive dyskinesia	Prolonged exposure to dopamine-blocking agents
Stimulant-induced chorea	Amphetamine or methylphenidate use
Anticonvulsant-induced chorea	Administration of phenytoin, phenobarbital, carbamazepine, or ethosuximide
Levodopa-induced chorea	Chorea in "on" periods of patients with Parkinson's disease treated with dopaminergic agents
Spontaneous dyskinesia	Oral-buccal lingual dyskinesia in elderly patients

Note. ANA = antinuclear antibody. CT = computed tomography.
MRI = magnetic resonance imaging. SLE = systemic lupus erythematosus.
T_4 = thyroxine. TSH = thyroid-stimulating hormone.

may occur if the patient is able to remain off dopamine-blocking agents for 1–2 years. The disorder may be permanent, and failure to resolve is particularly common in elderly patients. TD is suppressed by reintroducing or increasing the dose of dopamine-blocking drugs. It may improve with treatment with reserpine, propranolol, or clonazepam. A syndrome identical to TD may occur in elderly patients with no history of exposure to dopamine-blocking agents.

CHOREA WITH SYSTEMIC LUPUS ERYTHEMATOSUS

Chorea may occur in systemic lupus erythematosus (SLE). Chorea is most common in women whose disease begins early (around age 18 years). It is most frequent in SLE patients who have anti-phospholipid antibodies and may also occur in patients with anti-phospholipid antibodies who lack other evidence of SLE. Recurrent bouts of hemichorea and asymmetric chorea are common. SLE may be complicated by a variety of neuropsychiatric disorders including psychosis, depression, and seizures. The diagnosis of SLE is supported by a positive antinuclear antibody (ANA) test and, more specifically, by a positive anti-double-stranded DNA test. Antiphospholipid antibodies include lupus anticoagulant and anticardiolipin A and B.

SYDENHAM'S CHOREA AND CHOREA GRAVIDARUM

Sydenham's chorea follows group A streptococcal infections, although the original episode may not be recognized clinically. The chorea typically begins 1–6 months after the original infection. It is a small-amplitude chorea affecting primarily the distal muscles (hands and fingers). Sedimentation rate and antistreptolysin O titer may be normal; a test for anti-DNase B is usually positive. The chorea typically resolves in 4–6 months but may occasionally persist. Sydenham's chorea is accompanied by irritability, and both the acute and the postchoreic states may be associated with obsessional and compulsive symptoms.

Most patients who exhibit chorea during pregnancy (chorea gravidarum) or when taking oral contraceptives have a previous history of Sydenham's chorea, and these disorders represent reactivation of a latent movement disorder.

■ DYSTONIC DISORDERS

Dystonia refers to sustained muscle contraction that results in slow contortions or a continuously sustained abnormal posture. In the early stages of a dystonic disorder, the dystonia may occur only when using the involved limb, and intermittent muscle contraction may result in an action tremor. Dystonia may involve any muscles and may affect a single body part (focal dystonia), adjacent body parts (segmental dystonia), or essentially all muscle groups (generalized dystonia). Hereditary dystonia often begins in childhood. The onset is in the legs, and it progresses gradually to affect all body regions. Spontaneous remissions are not uncommon. Adult-onset idiopathic dystonia is usually focal or segmental, involving the neck (torticollis), jaw and eyelids (Meige's syndrome), or hand during writing (writer's cramp). Dystonia accompanies many choreic and parkinsonian syndromes (e.g., HD, PD), and tardive dystonia frequently co-occurs with TD.

No neuropsychiatric disorders are commonly associated with idiopathic dystonia, although the patients are often misdiagnosed as suffering from conversion disorders when the illness first begins.

■ TIC SYNDROMES

Tourette syndrome (TS) is one of several tic disorders (Table 10–4). It is characterized by onset of body and vocal tics before age 18 years. The tics wax and wane over time and persist throughout life. The components of the tic syndrome also vary over time, changing from one location to another and varying in complexity. The vocal tics may be unformed (e.g., throat clearing, sniffing) or formed (words); coprolalia (cursing) occurs in fewer than 50% of patients. There are no imaging or laboratory abnormalities in TS. Neuropathologic studies suggest that there is an increased number of dopamine receptors in the caudate nucleus and putamen. The tics can usually be suppressed by neuroleptic agents (e.g., haloperidol, pimozide), and some patients improve with clonidine or clonazepam.

Two principal neuropsychiatric disorders accompany TS: attention-deficit/hyperactivity disorder (ADHD) in childhood and OCD. ADHD occurs in approximately half of all TS patients in childhood, and TS sometimes first becomes evident when the child with ADHD is treated with stimulants and tics are precipitated. OCD occurs in approximately half of all TS patients and typically responds to treatment with conventional anti-OCD agents such as clomipramine and fluvoxamine. Self-mutilation and exhibitionism are occasional manifestations of OCD. In some families, OCD and TS are inherited in an autosomal-dominant manner, with some members having OCD, others manifesting TS, and some evidencing both disorders.

TABLE 10–4. **Classification of tic syndromes**

Idiopathic tic disorders
  Tourette syndrome
  Chronic multiple motor tic or phonic tic disorder
  Chronic single tic disorder
  Transient tic disorder
  Nonspecific tic disorder
Symptomatic tic disorders
  Postrheumatic tics (after rheumatic fever)
  Carbon monoxide exposure
  Neurodegenerative syndromes
    Neuroacanthocytosis
    Lesch-Nyhan syndrome
  Drug-induced tics
    Tardive tic disorders
    Stimulants (amphetamines, methylphenidate)
    Levodopa
    Anticonvulsants (phenytoin, carbamazepine, phenobarbital)

More limited idiopathic tic syndromes may occur in childhood or adulthood. Clinically, these syndromes are manifested by single or multiple tics without vocalizations. The tics are stable and unchanging over time. Tics may also be induced by a variety of drugs and can co-occur with other movement disorders (Table 10–4).

■ TREMOR

Tremors have no specific neuropsychiatric associations, but they may be induced by drugs that are commonly used in neuropsychiatry. Table 10–5 lists the features of two major types of tremor and their etiologies and treatment.

TABLE 10–5.   Characteristics of tremors (cerebellar intention-type tremors not included)

Characteristic	Rest tremor	Action tremor
Amplitude	Large	Small
Frequency	4–6 cps	10–12 cps
Present at rest	Yes	No
Increased by action	No	Yes
Reduced by alcohol	No	Yes
Increased by stress	Yes	Yes
Associated disorders	Parkinson's disease and parkinsonism	Benign essential tremor, tremor associated with dystonia, exaggerated physiologic tremor
Drugs that induce the tremor	Neuroleptics	Lithium, tricyclic antidepressants, stimulants, ephedrine, caffeine, valproate
Treatment	Reduce dosage of neuroleptic, administer anticholinergic or dopaminergic agents	Propranolol, primidone, clonazepam

Note.   cps = cycles per second.

■ CATATONIA

Catatonia is a complex motor disorder that occurs in psychiatric, neurologic, medical, and drug-induced conditions (Table 10–6). Catatonia includes a variety of movement disorders such as stereotypy (repetitive non-goal-directed movements), mannerisms (repetitive goal-oriented but bizarre or exaggerated movements),

TABLE 10–6. **Etiologies of catatonia**

Psychiatric disorders
  Depression
  Mania
  Schizophrenia
Neurologic disorders
  Encephalitis (especially herpes encephalitis)
  Subacute sclerosing panencephalitis
  General paresis
  Parkinson's disease
  Globus pallidus lesions
  Thalamic infarction
  Medial frontal infarctions or hemorrhage
  Epilepsy
Systemic disorders
  Diabetic ketoacidosis
  Hypercalcemia
  Hepatic encephalopathy
  Uremia
  Thrombocytopenic purpura
  Systemic lupus erythematosus
  Mononucleosis
Drug induced
  Amphetamines
  Phencyclidine (PCP)
  Neuroleptics
  Neuroleptic malignant syndrome

TABLE 10–7. **Neuroleptic-induced movement disorders**

Movement disorder	Clinical features
Acute dystonia	Onset 12–36 hours after starting or increasing neuroleptic; jaw, tongue, or trunk dystonia or oculogyric crises; relieved by anticholinergics or benzodiazepine
Akathisia	Onset 1–3 days after starting or increasing neuroleptic; restlessness; relieved by anti-cholinergic or propranolol
Akinesia	Onset 1–3 months after starting or increasing neuroleptic; slowness in initiating movements, diminished gesturing, reduced arm swing while walking; relieved by anticholinergics or amantadine
Parkinsonism	Onset 1–3 months after starting or increasing neuroleptic; rigidity and bradykinesia most common; relieved by anticholinergics or amantadine
Rest tremor	Occasionally the sole manifestation of drug-induced parkinsonism
Rabbit syndrome	Perioral tremor; part of the parkinsonian syndrome
TD	Onset after a minimum of 3 months of treatment; oral-lingual dyskinesia; poorly responsive to treatment; made worse by anticholinergics
Tardive dystonia	Common variant of TD; torticollis, blepharospasm, and jaw dystonia (Meige's syndrome) are most common; sometimes relieved by high-dose anticholinergics; best response is to local botulinum toxin injections
Tardive akathisia	An uncommon variant of TD; restless movements with less subjective distress than acute akathisia
Tardive tics	A rare variant of TD; involuntary tics
Tardive Tourette syndrome	A rare variant of TD; involuntary tics and vocalizations
Tardive myoclonus	A rare variant of TD; involuntary random jerking
Neuroleptic malignant syndrome	Rigidity, obtundation, fever, and autonomic abnormalities; elevated creatine phosphokinase

Note. TD = tardive dyskinesia.

sustained postures, waxy flexibility, catatonic unresponsiveness, automatic obedience, echolalia, and echopraxia. Treatment with benzodiazepines may be helpful and sometimes produces dramatic relief. Electroconvulsive therapy (ECT) is usually beneficial as well.

■ NEUROLEPTIC-INDUCED MOVEMENT DISORDERS

Several of the disorders discussed in this chapter can be induced by dopamine-blocking drugs. The widespread use of neuroleptic-type dopamine-blocking agents to treat psychotic and agitated patients results in a plethora of drug-induced movement abnormalities of which the clinician must be aware. Table 10–7 summarizes the major neuroleptic-induced movement disorders.

■ REFERENCES AND RECOMMENDED READING

Cummings JL: Clinical Neuropsychiatry. New York, Grune & Stratton, 1985

Cummings JL: Intellectual impairment in Parkinson's disease: clinical, pathologic, and biochemical correlates. J Geriatr Psychiatry Neurol 1:24–36, 1988

Cummings JL: Behavioral complications of drug treatment in Parkinson's disease. J Am Geriatr Soc 39:708–716, 1991

Cummings JL: Depression in Parkinson's disease. Am J Psychiatry 149:443–454, 1992

de Bruin VMS, Lees AJ: The clinical features of 67 patients with clinically definite Steele-Richardson-Olszewski syndrome. Behavioural Neurology 5:229–232, 1992

Folstein SE: Huntington's Disease: A Disorder of Families. Baltimore, MD, Johns Hopkins University Press, 1989

Frankel M, Cummings JL, Robertson MM, et al: Obsessions and compulsions in Gilles de la Tourette's syndrome. Neurology 36:378–382, 1986

Grafton ST, Mazziotta JC, Pahl JJ, et al: A comparison of neurological, metabolic, structural, and genetic evaluations in persons at risk for Huntington's disease. Ann Neurol 28:614–621, 1990

Joseph AB, Young RR (eds): Movement Disorders in Neurology and Psychiatry. Boston, MA, Blackwell Scientific Publications, 1992

Koller WC (ed): Handbook of Parkinson's Disease, 2nd Edition. New York, Marcel Dekker, 1992

Lees AJ: Tics and Related Disorders. New York, Churchill Livingstone, 1985

Mayeux R, Denaro J, Hemenegildo N, et al: A population-based investigation of Parkinson's disease with and without dementia. Arch Neurol 49:492–497, 1992

Menza M, Harris D: Benzodiazepines and catatonia: an overview. Biol Psychiatry 26:842–846, 1989

Rogers D: Motor Disorder in Psychiatry. New York, Wiley, 1992

Taylor MA: Catatonia: a review of a behavioral neurologic syndrome. Neuropsychiatry, Neuropsychology, and Behavioral Neurology 3:48–72, 1990

The Tourette Syndrome Classification Study Group: Definitions and classification of tic disorders. Arch Neurol 50:1013–1016, 1993

Trimble M: Psychopathology and movement disorders: a new perspective on the Gilles de la Tourette syndrome. J Neurol Neurosurg Psychiatry (suppl):90–95, 1989

Weiner WJ, Lang AE: Movement Disorders: A Comprehensive Survey. Mount Kisco, NY, Futura Publishing, 1989

Weiner WJ, Lang AE (eds): Drug-Induced Movement Disorders. Mount Kisco, NY, Futura Publishing, 1992

Wirshing WC, Cummings JL: Tardive movements disorders. Neuropsychiatry, Neuropsychology, and Behavioral Neurology 3:23–35, 1990

STROKE AND BRAIN TUMORS

Cerebrovascular disease is one of the most common causes of acquired behavior change in adults. With the marked expansion of the cerebral cortex that occurred in human evolution, the cerebral vasculature was stretched and contorted, creating border zones and end arterial zones with little collateral circulation and a consequent vulnerability to ischemic injury. Moreover, the lateralization of cognitive functions in humans reduced redundancy and further increased the chance of intellectual dysfunction with focal lesions. These two themes in human evolution converge to make the brain vulnerable to ischemic injury and create a high likelihood of disability after stroke.

Tumors are a less common but important source of neurologic disability and behavior change in both adults and children. This chapter describes common stroke syndromes and their behavioral correlates and discusses brain tumors and their associated neuropsychiatric morbidity.

■ CEREBROVASCULAR DISEASE AND STROKE

TYPES OF CEREBROVASCULAR DISEASE

In the U.S. population, there are approximately 400,000 new strokes annually, and the total number of stroke victims in the nation is 1.7 million. Stroke is an age-related disorder, becoming increasingly common among older individuals. The annual incidence of stroke rises from approximately 100 per 100,000 among 45- to 54-year olds to approximately 2,000 per 100,000 in those over age 75 years. Men are at greater risk for stroke than women (1.33:1 ratio). Seventy percent of stroke survivors have a permanent occupational disability, and approximately 25% have vascular dementia.

There are several major types of stroke syndromes (Table 11–1). Atherothrombotic occlusions result from atherosclerotic (large vessels) or arteriosclerotic (arterioles) in situ obstruction of cerebral vessels. Cerebral emboli arise from the heart and are carried distally in the arterial circulation to the brain. Emboli occasionally arise from plaques in the carotid, vertebral, basilar arteries. Intracerebral hemorrhage is typically associated with hypertension and rupture of small aneurysms on the arterioles in the deep gray nuclei of the brain. Subarachnoid hemorrhage results from rupture of congenital aneurysms of the circle of Willis at the base of the brain. Transient ischemic attacks (TIAs) are produced by temporary interruption of the blood supply to the brain, usually from disease of the carotid arteries. TIAs occasionally occur with occlusion of small vessels and mark the occurrence of a lacunar infarction in deep brain structures.

The type of stroke syndrome observed clinically depends on the size of the cerebral vessel involved. Occlusion of the carotid arteries usually leads to a border-zone infarction at the junction of the middle cerebral artery territory with the territories of the anterior and posterior cerebral arteries or an infarction in the combined territories of the middle and anterior cerebral arteries. Occlusion of a stem or surface branch of the anterior, middle, or posterior cerebral artery produces a regional syndrome (aphasia, aprosodia, homonymous hemianopsia, etc.). Occlusion of the proximal

TABLE 11–1. **Relative frequency of types of stroke syndromes**

Syndrome	Frequency (%)
Atherothrombotic vascular occlusion	60
Cerebral embolus	15
Intracerebral hemorrhage	5
Subarachnoid hemorrhage	10
Transient ischemic attacks	7
Other	3

Ischemic Strokes

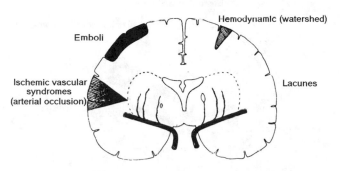

FIGURE 11–1. Locations of ischemic strokes. *Source.* Reprinted from Hachinski V, Norris JW: *The Acute Stroke.* Philadelphia, PA, FA Davis, 1985, p. 98. Used with permission.

branches of the intracerebral vessels that supply the basal ganglia, thalamus, and deep white matter produces lacunar infarctions and white matter ischemic injury. Vertebral or basilar compromise produces brain stem and posterior cerebral artery signs (nystagmus, dysarthria, diplopia, etc.). Figures 11–1 and 11–2 illustrate the locations of typical ischemic and hemorrhagic strokes, respectively.

RISK FACTORS FOR CEREBROVASCULAR DISEASE

The most potent risk factor for stroke is hypertension. Congestive heart failure, coronary artery disease, and electrocardiographic abnormalities are also highly correlated with stroke occurrence. Elevated blood lipids, cigarette smoking, diabetes, obesity, and elevated hematocrit also contribute to stroke risk. Cerebral emboli arise from the heart as a consequence of valvular disease, myocardial infarction with mural thrombus, cardiac arrhythmia (particularly atrial fibrillation), and cardiac surgery.

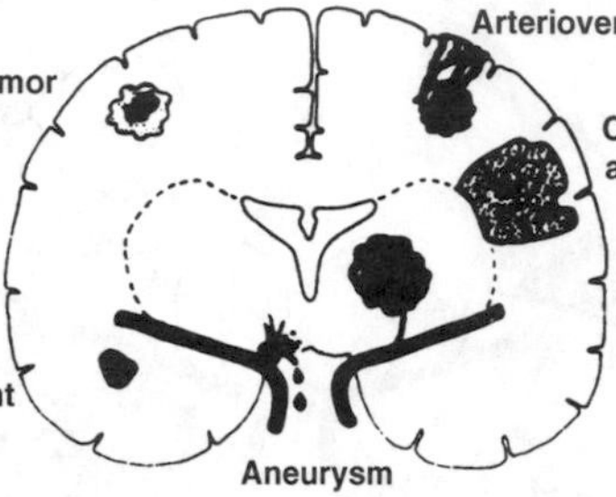

FIGURE 11–2. Locations of hemorrhagic strokes. *Source.* Reprinted from Hachinski V, Norris JW: *The Acute Stroke.* Philadelphia, PA, FA Davis, 1985, p. 98. Used with permission.

Among younger patients, a history of migraine and use of oral contraceptives are risk factors for stroke. Nonatherosclerotic vascular disorders such as collagen vascular diseases are also more common in younger stroke victims. Table 11–2 provides a list of disorders to be considered in younger individuals who have a stroke syndrome.

ASSESSMENT OF THE STROKE PATIENT

Evaluation of the stroke patient should include a complete blood count, prothrombin time and partial thromboplastin time (PT and PTT), erythrocyte sedimentation rate, electrolytes, blood sugar, blood urea nitrogen, serum cholesterol, electrocardiogram, and computed tomography (CT) or magnetic resonance imaging (MRI). Patients who sustain strokes but have no identifiable risk factors or who have a history of spontaneous abortions or migraine should be studied for the antiphospholipid antibody syndrome by obtaining anticardiolipin antibodies. Patients with TIAs may be

TABLE 11–2. **Etiologies of stroke in young individuals**

Systemic disorders
  Hypertension
  Diabetes
Cardiac disorders
  Rheumatic heart disease
  Prosthetic mitral valve
  Atrial myxoma
  Mitral valve prolapse
  Marantic endocarditis
  Atrial fibrillation
  Cardiomyopathy
  Patent foramen ovale
Trauma
  Carotid artery dissection
Vasculitis
  Systemic lupus erythematosus
  Antiphospholipid antibody
    syndrome
  Polyarteritis nodosa
  Behçet's disease
  Sarcoidosis
  Disseminated intravascular
    coagulation
  Thrombotic thrombocytopenic
    purpura
  Sneddon's syndrome
    (seronegative vasculitis with
    livido reticularis)
  Takayasu's disease
  Granulomatous angiitis
  Microangiopathy of retina and
    brain

Medication and drug induced
  Oral contraceptives
  Ergot derivatives
  Cocaine (oral or intravenous)
  Heroin (intravenous)
  Talwin (intravenous)
  Ritalin (intravenous)
Hematologic disorders
  Sickle-cell disease
  Polycythemia vera
  Leukemia with leukocytosis
  Hypercoagulation (idiopathic or
    with systemic cancer)
  Waldenström's
    macroglobulinemia
  Dysproteinemias
Infectious arteritis
  Syphilis
  Chronic basal meningitis
Inherited metabolic defects
  Homocystinuria
  Fabry's disease
  Mitochondrial encephalopathy
Cerebral venous thrombosis
  (may occur during
  pregnancy)
Migraine
Arteriovenous malformation
Fibromuscular dysplasia
Moya-Moya disease
Ehlers-Danlos syndrome
Pseudoxanthoma elasticum
Neoplastic angioendotheliosis

candidates for carotid endarterectomy and should have Doppler studies of the carotid arteries or angiography. Echocardiography may be necessary to identify a source of emboli within the heart. Single photon emission computed tomography (SPECT) and positron-emission tomography (PET) usually reveal areas of diminished cerebral perfusion or metabolism larger than the areas of structural change demonstrated by CT or MRI.

TREATMENT OF CEREBROVASCULAR DISEASE

Acutely, the patient should be managed by maintaining blood pressure in the high-normal range and providing anticoagulation therapy if the stroke is evolving or if the stroke is small and is thought to have resulted from a cardiac embolus. Long-term anticoagulation therapy should be provided for patients with cardiac disorders such as atrial fibrillation. Other patients with atherothrombotic strokes should be treated with aspirin. Those who are intolerant of aspirin or who have additional strokes despite aspirin should be considered for treatment with ticlopidine. Physical therapy, speech therapy, and occupational therapy will optimize the outcome.

NEUROPSYCHIATRIC SYNDROMES ASSOCIATED WITH STROKE

The neuropsychiatric consequences of a stroke depend on the location and extent of the brain injury, the existence of other ischemic damage, and the premorbid intellectual and emotional functioning of the individual. Stroke-related frontal lobe syndromes (Chapter 4), aphasia (Chapter 5), visuospatial disorders (Chapter 6), and memory disorders (Chapter 7) have been described. Vascular dementia is discussed in Chapter 9. This chapter emphasizes abnormalities of mood and emotional function after a stroke. Neuropsychiatric disorders may be accompanied by motor and sensory abnormalities, or they may be the only manifestations of ischemic brain injury. Emotional and cognitive disorders may coexist or may occur independently. Table 11–3 lists the major behavioral disorders that occur after a stroke.

Depression is the most common poststroke neuropsychiatric syndrome and occurs in 30%–50% of stroke victims within 2 years of the initial event. About half of the patients meet criteria for major depressive episode, and half have minor depression similar to dysthymic disorder. Major depression is not correlated with the degree of disability, whereas minor depression is more closely related to the patient's deficit syndrome. Depression is most common with lesions affecting the frontal lobes (dorsolateral prefrontal cortex and head of the caudate nucleus), and the frequency and severity of depression increase with increasing proximity of the lesion to the frontal pole. Lesions producing depression are more commonly found in the left frontal lobe than in the right frontal lobe; PET reveals bilateral frontal hypometabolism in patients who manifest a mood disorder. Anxiety accompanies cortical, but not subcortical, lesions that produce depression. Poststroke depression and anxiety respond to conventional psychotropic agents (Chapter 14). Several recent studies with MRI have found an increased prevalence of periventricular white matter lesions in patients with late-onset "idiopathic" depression. The changes may be vascular in

TABLE 11–3. **Principal behavioral alterations occurring after a stroke**

Neuropsychiatric disorders	Cognitive disorders
Depression	Aphasia
Mania	Executive dysfunction
Anxiety	Aprosodia
Apathy	Memory impairment
Psychosis	Constructional disturbances
Hallucinations	Unilateral neglect
Anosognosia	
Catastrophic reaction	
Emotional lability	

origin, suggesting that the associated depression is a manifestation of subtle ischemic brain injury.

Mania is much less common than depression after a stroke. It occurs almost exclusively with lesions of the right hemisphere. The lesions may affect the inferior medial frontal cortex, caudate nucleus, thalamus, or basal temporal region. Many of the patients have a family history of affective disorder. Cortical lesions produce single manic events; subcortical lesions may initiate a series of relapsing depressive and manic episodes similar to those of idiopathic bipolar disorder. Lithium and carbamazepine are the most efficacious antimanic medications (Chapter 14).

Psychosis is a rare complication of single strokes; it may occur with lesions of the left temporal region producing Wernicke's aphasia, with lesions of the right temporoparietal region, and with subcortical lesions affecting the caudate nuclei. Right-sided lesions are often accompanied by visual hallucinations and delusions. Seizures are common in patients who manifest poststroke psychosis. Psychosis is more common with bilateral cerebrovascular lesions. Poststroke delusions are treated with traditional antipsychotic agents (Chapter 14).

Visual hallucinations occur with retinal ischemia in amaurosis fugax, optic nerve lesions in ischemic optic neuritis, midbrain lesions in the syndrome of peduncular hallucinosis, and lesions of the geniculocalcarine radiations that produce homonymous visual-field defects ("release" hallucinations). Stroke-related seizures of the temporal, parietal, or occipital cortex may produce visual hallucinations. *Auditory hallucinations* may occur with pontine or temporal lobe ischemic injuries and may accompany poststroke delusions.

■ BRAIN TUMORS

Intracranial neoplasms can present with neuropsychiatric disturbances, or behavioral alterations may evolve as the tumor enlarges. Detection of an underlying tumor is important because increased intracranial pressure can be life threatening and treatment of the tumor must be implemented. Some tumors are benign and can be removed completely, whereas others are malignant and subject only to palliative treatment.

TYPES OF BRAIN TUMORS

Table 11–4 presents the major types of brain tumors and the relative frequency of their occurrence. Gliomas arise from the nonneural central nervous system (CNS) cells lines, including astrocytes (gliomas, astrocytomas), arachnoid cells (meningiomas), ependymal cells (ependymomas), oligodendrocytes (oligodendrogliomas), and embryonic cerebellar cells (medulloblastomas). Gliomas and meningiomas usually occur around age 50 years; medulloblastoma occurs before age 20 years. Gliomas are the most malignant and the most common intracranial tumors. Survival after diagnosis rarely exceeds 2 years even with aggressive surgical management, radiation, and chemotherapy. Astrocytomas are much less malignant, and some patients survive for several decades. Meningiomas are benign tumors, although they

TABLE 11–4. Relative frequency of types of brain tumors	
Tumor type	**Frequency (%)**
Glioblastoma multiforme	20
Meningioma	15
Astrocytoma	10
Pituitary adenoma	7
Neurinoma	7
Metastatic tumors	6
Ependymoma	6
Oligodendroglioma	5
Medulloblastoma	4
Craniopharyngioma and related tumors	4
Other	16

may recur after surgical resection if removal is incomplete or if tumor fragments are left in place because of their proximity to critical structures. Medulloblastomas usually occur in the first decade of life and are highly radiosensitive. Metastases arise from carcinomatous tumors occurring in lung, breast, melanomas, gastrointestinal tract, and kidney (in decreasing order of frequency). Breast and prostate tumors and multiple myeloma often metastasize to the skull and dura. The discovery that the patient has more than one intracranial tumor favors the diagnosis of metastatic disease.

CLINICAL FEATURES OF BRAIN TUMORS

Headaches are prominent in one-third of patients with tumors. The headache is typically nonpulsatile and intermittent. Seizures are very common in conjunction with intracranial tumors, occurring in 30%–40% of patients with gliomas, 60%–70% of patients with astrocytomas, and up to half of patients with meningiomas. Increased intracranial pressure produces papilledema characterized by obscuration of the optic disk margins, disk hyperemia, retinal hemorrhages, cotton-wool spots, and venous engorgement. Vision is not affected by papilledema. Unilateral weakness, sensory loss, ataxia, or homonymous visual-field defects may be present depending on the location of the tumor.

NEUROPSYCHIATRIC SYNDROMES ASSOCIATED WITH BRAIN TUMORS

Tumors produce behavioral disturbances similar to those that occur with stroke (Table 11–3), but the syndromes are usually less discrete because neoplasms and their associated edema and increased intracranial pressure tend to produce more extensive dysfunction. Mental status changes characteristic of mild delirium with slowness of thought, reduced attention, and impaired comprehension are typical of patients with intracranial tumors. Irritability is also common. These symptoms may be combined with more focal symptoms such as aphasia. Meningiomas sometimes rise from the floor of the anterior cranial fossa, producing orbitofrontal compression and a progressive frontal lobe syndrome. Frontal lobe tumors are particularly likely to cause depression; temporal lobe tumors produce psychosis or atypical mood disturbances with euphoria, hypomania, and lability. Diencephalic tumors may cause hypomania.

TREATMENT

Steroids are used to reduce edema associated with intracranial tumors. The role of surgery, radiation therapy, and chemotherapy is dictated by the tumor type. Seizures are treated with carbamazepine, phenytoin, gabapentin, lamotrigine, or valproate. Behavioral disturbances are treated with conventional psychotropic agents (Chapter 14). Increased intracranial pressure is a contraindication to the use of electroconvulsive therapy.

■ REFERENCES AND RECOMMENDED READING

Adams RD, Victor M: Principles of Neurology, 5th Edition. New York, McGraw-Hill, 1993

Beckson M, Cummings JL: Neuropsychiatric aspects of stroke. Int J Psychiatry Med 21:1–15, 1991

Bornstein RA, Brown G (eds): Neurobehavioral Aspects of Cerebrovascular Disease. New York, Oxford University Press, 1991

Caplan LR, Stein RW: Stroke: A Clinical Approach. Boston, MA, Butterworths, 1986

Cascino GD, Adams RD: Brainstem auditory hallucinations. Neurology 36:1042–1047, 1986

Cummings JL, Miller BL: Visual hallucinations: clinical occurrence and use in differential diagnosis. West J Med 146:46–51, 1987

Gorman DG, Cummings JL: Neurobehavioral presentations of the antiphospholipid antibody syndrome. J Neuropsychiatry Clin Neurosci 5:37–42, 1993

Hachinski V, Norris JW: The Acute Stroke. Philadelphia, PA, FA Davis, 1985

Kolmel HW: Complex visual hallucinations in the hemianopic field. J Neurol Neurosurg Psychiatry 48:29–38, 1985

Lepore FE: Spontaneous visual phenomena with visual loss: 104 patients with lesions of retinal and neural afferent pathways. Neurology 40:444–447, 1990

McKee AC, Levine DN, Kowall NW, et al: Peduncular hallucinosis associated with isolated infarction of the substantia nigra pars reticulata. Ann Neurol 27:500–504, 1990

Robinson RG, Starkstein SE: Current research in affective disorders following stroke. J Neuropsychiatry Clin Neurosci 2:1–14, 1990

Starkstein SE, Robinson RG: Depression in cerebrovascular disease, in Depression in Neurologic Disease. Edited by Starkstein SE, Robinson RG. Baltimore, MD, Johns Hopkins University Press, 1993, pp 28–49

Starkstein SE, Robinson RG: Neuropsychiatric aspects of stroke, in Textbook of Geriatric Neuropsychiatry. Edited by Coffey EC, Cummings JL. Washington, DC, American Psychiatric Press, 1994, pp 457–477

Starkstein SE, Pearlson GD, Boston J, et al: Mania after brain injury. Arch Neurol 44:1069–1073, 1987

WHITE MATTER DISEASES AND INBORN ERRORS OF METABOLISM

Brain white matter is composed of the neuronal axons, the majority of which are myelinated. Myelin, which is composed of protein and several lipids such as cholesterol, lecithin, and cerebrosides, is formed in the central nervous system (CNS) by oligodendroglia. Several diseases destroy CNS myelin. These include *demyelinating* and *dysmyelinating* conditions. The loss of myelin leads to slowing down or blocking of action-potential conduction. The most prevalent demyelinating condition is *multiple sclerosis* (MS). Dysmyelinating conditions are mainly due to inborn errors of metabolism. Many hereditary diseases are now recognized to affect white matter, and the principal white matter diseases are listed in Table 12–1. In this chapter, the main disorders of gray matter storage are also discussed.

12

■ DEMYELINATING CONDITIONS

MULTIPLE SCLEROSIS

In MS, episodes of demyelination occur at various sites in the CNS. The destroyed areas are referred to as plaques. Pathologically, lymphocytes and astrocytes can be seen infiltrating the area of demyelination, with degraded myelin products but intact axons. The plaques are most common in the upper spinal cord, brain stem, and periventricular regions of the CNS. MRI studies have revealed that the plaques are often more diffuse than is suspected from clinical signs and symptoms. The relevance of these diffuse plaques to behavioral change is unclear.

TABLE 12–1.   **Disorders of demyelination and dysmyelination**

Demyelination

Ischemic

Binswanger's disease

Inflammatory

Multiple sclerosis

Postinfectious syndromes

Infections

Human immunodeficiency virus encephalopathy

Progressive multifocal leukoencephalopathy

Metabolic

Central pontine myelinolysis

Marchiafava-Bignami disease

Dysmyelination

Adrenoleukodystrophy (X linked)

Pelizaeus-Merzbacher disease (X-linked leukodystrophy without adrenal disease)

Metachromatic leukodystrophy (autosomal recessive)

Krabbe's disease (autosomal recessive)

Cerebrotendinous xanthomatosis

The cause of MS is unknown, but it is thought to be due to an infection acquired in childhood, in association with a genetic predisposition.

MS is diagnosed on the basis of evidence of multiple CNS white matter lesions, distributed in space and time. The onset is usually between ages 20 and 40 years, and characteristically the patient has relapses and remissions. In around 20% of patients, the disorder is slowly progressive.

Common presenting features are blurred vision, diplopia, vertigo, paresthesias, weakness, unsteadiness, incontinence, and impotence. Cerebellar signs are also common. There are no pathognomic signs, but *Lhermitte's symptom* (a brief sensation like an electric shock that occurs on flexing the neck) and heat sensitivity with increased disability in warm environments are often described.

Four clinical diagnostic syndromes are recognized: clinically probable, clinically definite, laboratory-supported probable, and laboratory-supported definite. The laboratory tests used are listed in Table 12–2, and the criteria for diagnosis are listed in Table 12–3. The cerebrospinal fluid (CSF) findings may include an increased number of mononuclear cells (>5/µl), mainly lymphocytes; increased protein; elevated concentrations of immunoglobulin G (IgG) and other immunoglobulins; and the presence of abnormal bands on CSF electrophoresis. These abnormal bands are called oligoclonal bands, and they represent IgG molecules of restricted heterogeneity. They are present in 90% of patients with MS. It is important to examine serum and CSF at the same time, because immunoglobulins can pass from serum into the CSF, and in MS, it is the intrathecal production of IgG that is important. The presence of oligoclonal bands, however, is not

TABLE 12–2. **Laboratory tests used in the diagnosis of multiple sclerosis (MS)**

Test	MS patients with abnormal test results (%)[a]
Cerebrospinal fluid	
Raised lymphocyte count	33
Increased immunoglobulin level	90
Oligoclonal bands	90
Evoked potentials	
Sensory	70–90
Visual	90
Brain stem	40–60
Magnetic resonance imaging	
High-signal lesion	90–95

[a]Percentages are approximate.

190

TABLE 12–3. **Criteria for diagnosis of multiple sclerosis subtypes**

Clinically definite
- Two attacks of neurologic symptoms, each lasting at least 24 hours and separated by at least 1 month, involving different areas of the nervous system
- Either clinical evidence of two separate lesions on physical examination or clinical evidence of one lesion and laboratory evidence of a separate lesion (e.g., an abnormal evoked response)

Laboratory-supported definite
- Two attacks, clinical or laboratory evidence of one lesion, and the presence of oligoclonal bands in the cerebrospinal fluid
- One attack, clinical evidence of one lesion and laboratory evidence of a separate lesion, and oligoclonal bands
- Progressive course for 6 months, sequential discrete involvement clinically or paraclinically, and the presence of oligoclonal bands

Clinically probable
- Two attacks and clinical evidence of one lesion
- One attack and clinical evidence of two lesions
- One attack, clinical evidence of one lesion, and laboratory evidence of a separate lesion

Laboratory-supported probable
- Two attacks and the presence of oligoclonal bands

specific for MS, and these bands can be found in other CNS infections and systemic conditions (e.g., systemic lupus erythematosus) that evoke immune reactions.

The neuropsychiatric consequences of MS are listed in Table 12–4. Initial presentation with psychiatric symptoms has been described, but it is rare. MS is one cause of dementia.

Minor psychiatric morbidity is common, and the lifetime prevalence for major depression is 40%–50%. Psychiatric symptoms may be associated with relapse. Occasionally, they may represent the chief manifestation of an episode of demyelination.

TABLE 12–4.	**Neuropsychiatric consequences of multiple sclerosis**
Cognitive impairment (common)	Euphoria
Memory disorder (common)	Emotional lability
Frank dementia (rare: 5%)	Delirium (rare)
Depression	Psychosis (rare)
Fatigue	Suicide

Stress has always been suggested as a factor that may precipitate relapse. Severely threatening life events are increased in MS patients compared with control subjects in the 6 months before disease onset.

A mental state consisting of euphoria (a cheerful complacency) and eutonia (a sense of bodily well-being) was earlier thought to be relatively specific for MS. It is now recognized that this picture is associated with intellectual decline, enlarged ventricles on computed tomography (CT), and probably with periventricular plaques. Emotional lability is also associated with periventricular plaques, especially in the frontal areas.

In contrast to some gray matter disorders such as epilepsy, psychoses are rare in MS. Recent magnetic resonance imaging (MRI) studies provide evidence that when they occur, delusions are associated with CNS plaques around the temporal horns of the lateral ventricles. Psychoses can also be precipitated by treatments, especially steroids.

There are no specific treatments to prevent or cure MS. Antispasticity drugs include benzodiazepines, baclofen, and dantrolene. Clonazepam or primidone may help the tremor. Adrenocorticotropic hormone (ACTH) and steroids are used to treat the acute episode of MS. Immunotherapy (azathioprine, cyclophosphamide, lymphoid irradiation, and plasma exchange) is used for the relapses. β-Interferon is of value in treating some patients.

LEUKOENCEPHALOPATHY

Patchy deep white matter lesions (unidentified bright objects [UBOs]) are often seen coincidentally on MRI T2-weighted scans. Past 60 years of age, UBOs are common (30%), and although they resemble lesions seen with infarction, their clinical significance is not yet known. However, they are increased in patients with depression and dementia. *Subcortical arteriosclerotic encephalopathy (Binswanger's disease)* is a vascular leukoencephalopathy that presents as a dementia (see Chapter 9).

Some deficiency states can lead to myelin destruction. Most notable are vitamin B_{12} and folic acid depletion. *Subacute combined degeneration* is the classic neurologic syndrome of B_{12} deficiency. This syndrome is associated with a megaloblastic anemia and usually with some disorder of the gastrointestinal tract or dietary insufficiency. It involves peripheral neuropathy and myelopathy. The cerebral manifestations of B_{12} deficiency range from mild forgetfulness and irritability to psychoses, confusional states, and dementia. Folate deficiency has been linked to depression, and mental retardation is a feature of some genetic disorders of folate metabolism.

CENTRAL PONTINE MYELINOLYSIS

Central pontine myelinolysis is a rare disorder in which the myelin sheaths in the pons are destroyed in a symmetrical manner. It may occur in alcoholism, states of malnutrition, and after electrolyte imbalance, especially low-sodium states. Often, subtle changes in mental state, dysarthria, and pseudobulbar palsy may be seen. In malnourished patients, central pontine myelinolysis may accompany Wernicke's encephalopathy.

MARCHIAFAVA-BIGNAMI SYNDROME

Another rare condition, which is secondary to alcoholism, that leads to progressive behavior changes and then dementia is the

Marchiafava-Bignami syndrome. There is selective demyelination of the corpus callosum, and the presentation is often as a frontal dementia.

■ DYSMYELINATING CONDITIONS

In dysmyelinating conditions, there is abnormal development of myelin due to inborn errors of metabolism. In general, the older that patients are at presentation, the more likely they will have psychiatric problems and the dysmyelinating condition will present as a psychiatric illness.

One of the more common leukodystrophies is *metachromatic leukodystrophy*. It is an autosomal-recessive disorder due to a deficiency of aryl-sulfatase A, leading to an accumulation of sulfated sphingolipids. There is central and peripheral demyelination. Patients with the juvenile and adult-onset forms present with behavioral symptoms, which include personality changes, dementia, and a schizophrenia-like illness.

Metachromatic granules can be found in the urine and the peripheral nerves, and the diagnosis of metachromatic leukodystrophy is confirmed by assessing the enzyme activity in leukocytes or fibroblasts. CT and MRI reveal central demyelination. Evoked potentials are abnormal, and nerve conduction times are slowed.

Adrenoleukodystrophy is an X-linked autosomal-recessive condition due to impairment of beta-oxidation of very long chain fatty acids. Usually males are affected. There is diffuse white matter demyelination, especially of the corticospinal tracts, and MRI reveals extensive white matter lesions. Dementia, learning difficulties, and behavior changes are the most frequent presenting psychiatric problems, but schizophrenia-like states have been reported. Adrenoleukodystrophy is best detected by direct measurement of saturated very long chain fatty acids in plasma. *Krabbe's disease* is an autosomal-recessive storage disorder with a buildup of galactocerebrosides (lipids) in macrophages in the white matter due to a deficiency of galactocerebrosidase. It is detected by assay of leukocytes or fibroblasts for the enzyme.

■ OTHER INBORN ERRORS OF METABOLISM

Other inborn errors of metabolism are a heterogeneous group of disorders in which abnormal metabolites accumulate in neurons or specific metabolites are deficient. Generally, these disorders lead to early death. However, some, like the leukoencephalopathies discussed above, have later ages of onset and present with slow onset of psychiatric symptoms, often in the form of a personality disorder or a psychosis, before leading to obvious dementia. Most are inherited as autosomal-recessive or X-linked conditions. The most important of these disorders are listed in Chapter 9, Table 9–8. There are many others—for example, *phenylketonuria,* which is due to accumulation of phenylalanine, and the *porphyrias,* in which the CNS changes are part of a more generalized metabolic encephalopathy. The former is due to a deficiency of the enzymes metabolizing phenylalanine, and there is an accumulation of phenylalanine in the blood. It is autosomal recessive and is usually detected by screening in the neonatal period. It is treated by a low-phenylalanine diet.

Nearly all of the mucopolysaccharidoses present in childhood. *Kufs disease* (late-onset neuronal ceroid lipofuscinoses) and several of the *sphingolipidoses* present later in life. The sphingolipidoses are subdivided in various groups. They include the *gangliosidoses,* Niemann-Pick disease, Krabbe's disease, and metachromatic leukodystrophy. There is obvious overlap here with the dysmyelinations. Diagnosis, if possible, requires either tissue biopsy or enzyme assays of leukocytes or fibroblasts.

■ REFERENCES AND
RECOMMENDED READING

Francis GS, Antel JP, Duquette P: Inflammatory demyelinating diseases of the CNS, in Neurology in Clinical Practice. Edited by Bradley WG,

Daroff RB, Fenichel GM, et al. Boston, MA, Butterworths, 1991, pp 1133–1166

Grant I, Brown G, Harris T, et al: Severely threatening events and marked life difficulties preceding onset or exacerbation of multiple sclerosis. J Neurol Neurosurg Psychiatry 52:8–13, 1989

Joffe RT, Lippert GP, Gray TA, et al: Mood disorder and multiple sclerosis. Arch Neurol 44:376–378, 1987

Kitchin W, Cohen-Cole SA, Mickel SF: Adrenoleukodystrophy: frequency of presentation as psychiatric disorder. Biol Psychiatry 22:1375–1387, 1987

Poser CM, Paty D, Scheinberg L, et al: New diagnostic criteria for multiple sclerosis. Ann Neurol 13:227–231, 1983

Rabins PV, Brooks BR, O'Donnell P, et al: Structural correlates of emotional disorders in multiple sclerosis. Brain 109:585–597, 1986

Ron MA: Multiple sclerosis and the mind. J Neurol Neurosurg Psychiatry 55:1–3, 1992

Ron MA, Logsdail SJ: Psychiatric morbidity in multiple sclerosis: a clinical and MRI study. Psychol Med 19:887–895, 1989

HEAD INJURY AND ITS SEQUELAE

The incidence of head injury in the United States is estimated to be between 175 and 367 per 100,000. Of these injuries, 7% may be considered severe. The most common causes are falls, road traffic accidents, and assaults. However, head injuries are not randomly distributed in the population. In the United States, 20% are due to the use of firearms, and semiskilled and unskilled workers are overrepresented, as are those who engage in substance abuse. Head injury accounts for 1% of all deaths but also leads to considerable morbidity. The morbidity depends on a number of factors, including the site and the severity of the injury, the premorbid status of the patient, and the presence or the absence of complications such as epilepsy.

13

There are several ways to assess the severity of a head injury. One commonly used method is the duration of posttraumatic amnesia (PTA) (see Chapter 7). Another is the depth of any coma, which is sometimes easier to gauge than the PTA. Several validated rating scales to assess head injury are in use (Table 13–1). The Glasgow Coma Scale assesses eye opening, verbal responses, and motor responses; higher scores correspond to less severe injury. A coma that lasts more than 6 hours indicates a severe injury.

The pathogenesis of the trauma is either direct or indirect. With direct trauma, an object or torn meninges or skull impinge on brain tissue. Effects include contusions and brain lacerations. Shearing forces injure the long white matter fibers, leading to diffuse axonal injury. The higher the velocity of the head injury, the more likely that shearing of white matter tracts occurs. Because the anterior poles of the frontal and temporal cortices are tightly held by the rigid anterior fossae of the skull, damage occurs preferentially at these sites. These poles are the areas most likely to show so-called contrecoup injuries.

TABLE 13–1.   **Scales used to assess head injury**

Length of posttraumatic amnesia

<5 min = very mild
≥5 min to <1 h = mild
≥1 h to <24 h = moderate
≥24 h to <1 wk = severe
≥1 wk = very severe

Glasgow Coma Scale[a]

Eye opening	Motor response	Verbal response
1. Nil	1. Nil	1. Nil
2. To pain	2. Extensor	2. Groans
3. To speech	3. Flexor	3. Inappropriate
4. Spontaneously	4. Withdrawal	4. Confused
	5. Localizing	5. Oriented
	6. Voluntary	

[a] 1–4 = very severe; 5–8 = severe; 9–12 = moderate; ≥13 = mild.

Indirect injury arises from shearing forces that lead to parenchymatous damage. This damage occurs in part because of rotational movements of the brain, which lag behind movements of the skull, setting up destructive intracranial forces. Where the glide of the brain inside the skull is greatest, small dural tears and bleeding of the surface blood vessels occur—usually in the parieto-occipital regions.

Other causes of indirect injury are cerebral bleeding and thrombosis, hypoxia, raised intracranial pressure, and herniation of brain tissue. The hippocampus is particularly affected by *transtentorial herniation*.

There is debate over the long-term consequences of boxing. The term *punch drunk* suggests that patients have dysarthria, ataxia, and cognitive changes. *Dementia pugilistica* is an alternative diagnosis. This state, which occurs after repeated sublethal blows to the brain, is associated with pathologic changes to the subcortical midline structures and cerebellum. Damage to the substantia nigra results in parkinsonism. At autopsy, patients with dementia pugilistica have abundant intracellular neurofibrillary tangles without Alzheimer-type neuritic plaques.

The most common neurologic complications of head injury are intracranial hematoma, infection, and epilepsy. The epilepsy is usually focal, but may present as a secondarily generalized seizure. The chances of developing epilepsy correlate with three factors: the length of the PTA, the presence or absence of an early seizure, and the presence or absence of a depressed skull fracture (Table 13–2).

Imaging studies are relevant for the assessment of head injury. Magnetic resonance imaging (MRI) may show intracranial lesions that are not revealed by computed tomography (CT), and perfusion deficits may be demonstrated by single photon emission computed tomography (SPECT). There is an association between persistent neuropsychological deficits and both ventricular dilation and deep white matter lesions on MRI.

TABLE 13–2. **Chances of developing late epilepsy after head injury**

Condition	Approx. chance of developing late epilepsy (%)
PTA >24 h + depressed fracture + early seizure	60–70
Early seizure + PTA >24 h	50
PTA >24 h + depressed fracture	30
Depressed fracture + early seizure	25
Depressed fracture	20
PTA >24 h	20
Early seizure	15

Note. More than half of head injury patients who develop posttraumatic epilepsy have a seizure within 1 year of their injury, and three-quarters have a seizure within 3 years. PTA = posttraumatic amnesia.

■ PERSONALITY CHANGES SECONDARY TO NEUROLOGIC INJURY

After head injury, three independent mechanisms operate to shape the resulting personality. These are the premorbid personality, a generalized cerebral disturbance, and the results of any focal deficits, especially frontal damage.

The premorbid personality may become exaggerated. An excessively tidy person may develop overt obsessional tendencies; a person with a sociopathic personality may manifest explosive violence.

The generalized deficits plus frontal lobe injury lead to a regular pattern of symptoms that are often subtle and at first may not be attributed to the underlying brain damage. They are listed in Table 13–3. In general, there is poor tolerance of environmental change, stimulus boundedness (the patient becomes more dependent on external stimuli for action), concretization and loss of mental flexibility, and affective change with irritability, lability, and explosiveness. With more severe damage, extremes of this profile are seen, with social disorganization, loss of interest in the self, explosive irritability, and a shallow, labile, blunted affect. These personality changes may be intertwined with the effects of

TABLE 13–3. **Generalized disturbance of cerebral function that may be seen after head trauma**

Activity influenced more by external stimuli	Posttraumatic orderliness
Impaired ability to use abstract concepts	Posttraumatic slovenliness
Concretization	Disturbed and labile affect
Disturbed attention and concentration	Psychomotor slowing
Disturbed spontaneity	Fatigability
Poverty of ideas	Memory complaints
	Diminished social awareness
	Indecision
	Loss of intellectual flexibility

focal damage and posttraumatic stress disorder (PTSD) (see below).

■ OTHER NEUROPSYCHIATRIC CONSEQUENCES OF TRAUMA

Cognitive changes are also both generalized and focal. There is blunting of overall performance on standardized IQ tests, with a decline from estimated premorbid levels. The patient's premorbid IQ is often assessed by using the educational history of the patient combined with a test of word reading ability such as the National Adult Reading Test. Focal deficits reflect those areas of the cortex that are directly damaged. Memory disturbance is common, with impaired learning of new material and slowing of retrieval. Psychomotor slowing (bradyphrenia) is common with more severe injury. These neurocognitive deficits may be compounded in patients with substance abuse and the continued use of alcohol.

Psychoses are not common. When they occur, they are schizophrenia-like, paranoid, or affective. These psychoses are more common with left-sided injuries, especially if the temporal lobes are involved. As in many organic psychotic states, affect may be preserved in the presence of a florid delusional disorder.

Mania is not frequent. It is more frequent after right-hemisphere (especially limbic) lesions.

Depression is common (20%–50%), and the clinical picture often is confounded by the features shown in Table 12–3. There is evidence that left dorsolateral frontal cortical lesions and left basal ganglia lesions are associated with major depression, more often than are lesions in other brain areas. Among causes of death, suicide is overrepresented, leading to 14% of all deaths.

POSTCONCUSSIONAL SYNDROME

The nosologic status of this condition is always in doubt. However, many patients who have had head injury complain of headache, dizziness, diplopia, fatigue, sensitivity to noise, and poor concentration. Most of the patients become asymptomatic within a few weeks of the injury. A small percentage remain symptomatic. In some patients, there may be signs of central nervous system (CNS) damage—for example, auditory evoked-potential changes, abnormal caloric tests, and acute vertigo and nystagmus on suddenly lying down. These symptoms may become persistent and blend in with those of anxiety, depression, and often PTSD.

There are several etiologic factors underlying the chronic nonpsychotic disorders of cerebral trauma (Table 13–4). The emotional impact of a head injury is variable. However, the head does hold a special place in the body image; consequently, head injury poses a threat that does not apply to other body parts. Furthermore, the circumstances of the accident may not be straightforward and may have personal consequences for patients, leading to unresolved conflict or guilt (e.g., when a friend or relative is killed).

The development of PTSD after head injury is common. The DSM-IV criteria are given in Table 13–5 (American Psychiatric Association 1994). It is partially true that the more severe the head injury, the less likely that PTSD will develop. This is because patients with marked brain damage are more likely to have an amnesia for the psychological trauma of the accident. However, many patients with severe head injuries have PTSD, but it is often

---

TABLE 13–4. **Some etiologic factors in psychiatric disturbance after head injury**

Mental constitution	Response to intellectual impairments
Premorbid personality	
Emotional impact of the injury	Epilepsy
Emotional repercussions of the injury	Amount of brain damage
	Location of brain damage
Environmental factors	History of substance abuse
Compensation and litigation	

Source. Adapted from Lishman 1987.

TABLE 13–5. **DSM-IV criteria for posttraumatic stress disorder**

A. The person has been exposed to a traumatic event in which both of the following were present:

1. The person experienced, witnessed, or was confronted with an event or events that involved actual or threatened death or serious injury, or a threat to the physical integrity of self or others

2. The person's response involved intense fear, helplessness, or horror. **Note:** In children, this may be expressed instead by disorganized or agitated behavior

B. The traumatic event is persistently reexperienced in one (or more) of the following ways:

1. Recurrent and intrusive distressing recollections of the event, including images, thoughts, or perceptions. **Note:** In young children, repetitive play may occur in which themes or aspects of the trauma are expressed.

2. Recurrent distressing dreams of the event. **Note:** In children, there may be frightening dreams without recognizable content.

3. Acting or feeling as if the traumatic event were recurring (includes a sense of reliving the experience, illusions, hallucinations, and dissociative flashback episodes, including those that occur on awakening or when intoxicated). **Note:** In young children, trauma-specific reenactment may occur.

4. Intense psychological distress at exposure to internal or external cues that symbolize or resemble an aspect of the traumatic event

5. Physiological reactivity on exposure to internal or external cues that symbolize or resemble an aspect of the traumatic event

C. Persistent avoidance of stimuli associated with the trauma and numbing of general responsiveness (not present before the trauma), as indicated by three (or more) of the following:

1. Efforts to avoid thoughts, feelings, or conversations associated with the trauma

2. Efforts to avoid activities, places, or people that arouse recollections of the trauma

3. Inability to recall an important aspect of the trauma

(continued)

TABLE 13–5.	**DSM-IV criteria for posttraumatic stress disorder** *(continued)*

	4.	Markedly diminished interest or participation in significant activities
	5.	Feeling of detachment or estrangement from others
	6.	Restricted range of affect (e.g., unable to have loving feelings)
	7.	Sense of a foreshortened future (e.g., does not expect to have a career, marriage, children, or a normal life span)
D.		Persistent symptoms of increased arousal (not present before the trauma), as indicated by two (or more) of the following:
	1.	Difficulty falling or staying asleep
	2.	Irritability or outbursts of anger
	3.	Difficulty concentrating
	4.	Hypervigilance
	5.	Exaggerated startle response
E.		Duration of the disturbance (symptoms in Criteria B, C, and D) is more than 1 month.
F.		The disturbance causes clinically significant distress or impairment in social, occupational, or other important areas of functioning.

Specify if:

Acute: if duration of symptoms is less than 3 months

Chronic: if duration of symptoms is 3 months or more

Specify if:

With delayed onset: if onset of symptoms is at least 6 months after the stressor

Source. Reprinted from American Psychiatric Association: *Diagnostic and Statistical Manual of Mental Disorders,* 4th Edition. Washington, DC, American Psychiatric Association, 1994. Used with permission.

overlooked in the setting of much more obvious cognitive and physical changes.

Other posttraumatic syndromes include posttraumatic anxiety, with or without phobias and panic attacks; posttraumatic conversion disorder (including pseudoseizures); and posttraumatic obsessional states.

In a setting where financial compensation is involved, the possibility of *malingering* must be considered. There are no diagnostic tests useful to identify malingering.

The management of the behavioral complications of head injury is complicated and requires a multidisciplinary approach. Any substance abuse must be stopped, and psychotropic drugs should be used with care. Seizures are an ever-present risk, and many psychotropic drugs can cause convulsions. Behavioral techniques, cognitive retraining, and psychotherapy all form part of remedial therapy. In more severely disabled patients, the relatives and caregivers usually need help and support to cope with the changed personality and behavior of the injured person.

■ REFERENCES AND RECOMMENDED READING

American Psychiatric Association: Diagnostic and Statistical Manual of Mental Disorders, 4th Edition. Washington, DC, American Psychiatric Association, 1994

Corsellis JAN: Boxing and the brain. Br Med J 298:105–109, 1989

Federoff JP, Starkstein SE, Forrester AW, et al: Depression in patients with head injury. Am J Psychiatry 149:918–923, 1992

Goldstein K: After Effects of Brain Injuries in War. New York, Grune & Stratton, 1942

Jennett B, Teasdale G: Assessment of head injuries, in Management of Head Injuries (Contemporary Neurological Series). Philadelphia, PA, FA Davis, 1981, pp 301–316

Jorge RE, Robinson RG, Starkstein SE, et al: Depression and anxiety following traumatic brain injury. J Neuropsychiatry Clin Neurosci 5:369–374, 1993

Kraus JF: Epidemiology of head injury, in Head Injury, 2nd Edition. Edited by Cooper P. Baltimore, MD, Williams & Wilkins, 1987, pp 1–19

Levin HS, Benton AL, Grossman RG: Neurobehavioral Consequences of Head Injury. New York, Oxford University Press, 1982

Lishman WA: Organic Psychiatry, 2nd Edition. Oxford, England, Blackwell Scientific, 1987, pp 137–186

Starkstein SE, Pearlson GD, Boston J, et al: Mania after head injury. Arch Neurol 44:1069–1073, 1987

TREATMENTS IN NEUROPSYCHIATRY

All treatments in neurology and psychiatry exert their effect by alteration of brain function. This altered function is largely achieved by changes in neurotransmitters or their receptors, although in neurosurgical procedures, this alteration is effected by the placement of structural lesions. Neurologists and psychiatrists use a similar spectrum of drugs.

■ NEUROPSYCHOPHARMACOLOGY

BASIC CONCEPTS

The *bioavailability* of a drug is the proportion of an oral dose that reaches its site of action. Intravenous drugs have an assumed 100% bioavailability. The *clearance* of a drug is the volume of plasma cleared of that drug in a unit of time. Some drugs, when given orally, are partially metabolized by the gut and liver, the *first-pass effect*. The *half-life* of a drug is the time taken for its concentration to fall by 50%. With *first-order* kinetics, there is a linear relationship between the dose taken and the serum drug levels. In *second-order* kinetics, the relationship is curvilinear (see Figure 14–3). The *steady state* defines that circumstance in which the amount absorbed equals the amount eliminated, and plasma levels are stable. Steady state is usually achieved after five half-lives.

For most of the psychotropic agents discussed in this chapter, convincing relationships between side effects and serum levels and between therapeutic effects and serum levels have not been shown. Reasons for monitoring serum levels are to check compliance and to detect patients who may be metabolizing a drug anomalously.

A classification system for the main psychotropic agents is shown in Table 14–1.

14

TABLE 14–1. **Classification system for psychotropic drugs**

Antidepressants	**Psychostimulants**
MAOIs (MAO-A, MAO-B)	Methylphenidate
Non-MAOIs	Dextroamphetamine
Tricyclics	Pemoline
Nontricyclics[a]	**Mood-stabilizing drugs**
Major tranquilizers	Lithium
Phenothiazines	Others[b]
Butyrophenones	**Nootropics**
Atypical neuroleptics	Tacrine
Minor tranquilizers	**Others**
Barbiturates	β-Blockers
Benzodiazepines	Narcotics
Buspirone	Analgesics
	Dopamine agonists

Note. MAOIs = monoamine oxidase inhibitors.
[a]Nontricyclics include the selective serotonin reuptake inhibitors and others.
[b]Other mood-stabilizing drugs include anticonvulsants, valproic acid, and carbamazepine.

■ ANTIDEPRESSANTS

Monoamine oxidase inhibitors (MAOIs) act by inhibiting the activity of both the A and B forms of monoamine oxidase (MAO), an enzyme widely distributed throughout the body. The substrates for MAO-A include norepinephrine and serotonin; the substrate for MAO-B is phenylalanine. Tyramine and dopamine are substrates for both.

Selective inhibitors are available, including clorgyline and meclobemide, reversible inhibitors of MAO-A, and deprenyl, a reversible inhibitor of MAO-B.

The *cheese reaction* is due to an interaction between the inhibition of peripheral MAO activity and the ingestion of certain primary amines. This reaction produces hypertension after patients eat certain foods, and it is one of the reasons these drugs are not widely used. However, with the newer, selective drugs (e.g., meclobemide), this reaction is much less likely to occur.

Symptoms most likely to respond to MAOIs in clinical practice are listed in Table 14–2.

Deprenyl may play a neuroprotective role in Parkinson's disease due to its ability to reduce the generation of free radicals. *Free radicals* are intermediaries in the normal reductive process of molecular oxygen that generates high-energy phosphate compounds. These molecules have single unpaired electrons, are unstable, and oxidize neighboring molecules. Free radicals can lead to tissue damage—for example, by interacting with polyunsaturated lipids, which results in cell membrane injury. There exists a series of natural defense mechanisms, such as free-radical scavengers (ascorbate) and enzymes such as superoxide dismutase. Dopamine neurons may be especially vulnerable to oxidative stress through reactions catalyzed by MAO. A partial loss of neurons leads to increased turnover in the remaining cells, increasing free-radical formation and leading to further cell damage. Deprenyl may delay the progression of disability by reducing free-radical generation and ameliorating neurotoxicity.

The *tricyclic antidepressants* are traditionally thought to act by inhibiting monoamine uptake from the synaptic cleft. Drugs such as maprotiline, desipramine, and protriptyline are more selective for norepinephrine uptake, and clomipramine is more selective

---

TABLE 14–2. **Symptoms most likely to respond to monoamine oxidase inhibitors**

MAO-A inhibitors	MAO-B inhibitors
Atypical depression	Parkinson's disease
Somatic anxiety	
Agoraphobia and social phobias	
Phobic anxiety with depersonalization	
Atypical facial pain	

Note. MAO = monoamine oxidase.

for serotonin (5-HT). Anticholinergic effects are common, especially with amitriptyline and clomipramine. Several tricyclic antidepressants have antihistaminic properties, and a common effect of all antidepressant treatment (including electroconvulsive therapy [ECT]) is to downregulate the activity of β-adrenergic receptors.

The *selective serotonin reuptake inhibitors* (SSRIs) include fluoxetine, fluvoxamine, paroxetine, sertraline, and citalopram. They have fewer side effects than tricyclics and are safer in overdose.

The side effects of the non-MAOI antidepressants are shown in Table 14–3. The nausea, weight reduction, and tremor reported with the SSRIs probably reflect the serotonin uptake inhibition. One of the most problematic side effects is seizures. These occur at a rate of around 1 per 1,000 prescriptions, but they are more common with maprotiline, mianserin, clomipramine, and bupropion (in higher doses). Seizures occur with the SSRIs, and all of these drugs should be prescribed carefully for patients with a

TABLE 14–3. **Side effects of non-MAOI antidepressants**

Sedation	Tremor
Dry mouth	Dyskinesias
Palpitations	Myopathy
EEG changes	Neuropathy
Blurred vision	Convulsions
Postural hypotension	Ataxia
Nausea, vomiting, GI upset	Delirium
Constipation	Transient hypomania
Glaucoma	Agitation, aggression
Urinary retention	Depersonalization
Anorgasmia, impotence	Impaired cognition
Paralytic ileus	Cholestatic jaundice
Galactorrhea	Weight gain
Sweating, fever	Rash

Note. EEG = electroencephalogram. GI = gastrointestinal.
MAOI = monoamine oxidase inhibitor.

lowered seizure threshold, starting with low doses and increasing them gradually. Patients taking hepatic enzyme–inducing agents have lower serum antidepressant levels because of increased metabolism and may need larger doses. Patients with *resistant depression* also sometimes need high doses (e.g., up to 200–300 mg of a tricyclic agent daily). Sedating agents, including clomipramine and amitriptyline, should be given mainly at night.

SSRIs inhibit the metabolism of some drugs, including tricyclic antidepressants, carbamazepine, and haloperidol.

The main use of antidepressants is in the management of depression. However, they are also used to treat migraine, panic disorder, obsessive-compulsive disorder, and narcolepsy (clomipramine is specific for *cataplexy*).

■ MAJOR TRANQUILIZERS

Like the tricyclic antidepressants, the phenothiazines have a tricyclic nucleus, and the two classes of drugs share many of the same side effects. The atypical neuroleptics include molindone, loxapine, sulpiride, remoxipride, risperidone, and clozapine. The distinguishing features of the major tranquilizers are that they are antipsychotic and block dopamine receptors. The atypical neuroleptics act preferentially on dopamine receptors outside the dorsal striatum, which gives them a different side effect profile. The most potent dopamine antagonist is benperidol; pimozide is the most specific for dopamine receptors. The phenothiazines also have a range of effects on the 5-HT, α-adrenergic, histaminic, and cholinergic receptors.

The major tranquilizers evoke extrapyramidal reactions (see Chapter 10, Table 10–7). The most common are the acute, agitated restlessness of *akathisia* and the lack of spontaneous movement of *akinesia*. The atypical neuroleptics including sulpiride (a selective D_2 antagonist), risperidone (a D_2 and 5-HT$_2$ antagonist), and clozapine (a D_1 and D_4 antagonist) are thought to be less likely to lead to extrapyramidal complications.

The main use of neuroleptics is to treat psychotic disorders, particularly schizophrenia, mania, and psychosis in neurologic disorders. They are used in the management of *Huntington's chorea, delirium, Tourette syndrome,* and *borderline personality disorder.* Their adverse effects require that their use be minimized when alternative therapies are available.

■ MINOR TRANQUILIZERS

Barbiturates are rarely used these days, although phenobarbitone is prescribed as an anticonvulsant, often on the grounds of cost. They are associated with *hyperactivity* and *attention-deficit/hyperactivity disorder* in children and depression in adults. They cause respiratory depression, leading to death in overdose.

The benzodiazepines have a common structure but a spectrum of activity that ranges from full agonist to antagonist to inverse agonist effects. Because of the variety of actions, they have tranquilizing, anticonvulsant, muscle-relaxant, and amnestic properties (producing memory impairments) (see Figure 14–1). They act at the benzodiazepine–γ-aminobutyric acid (GABA) receptor.

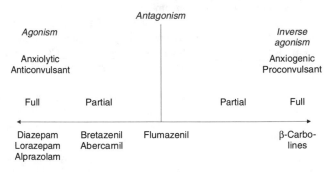

FIGURE 14–1. Spectrum of the effects of benzodiazepines.

TABLE 14–4. **Pharmacologic differences among benzodiazepines**

Long acting (tranquilizers)	Intermediate acting (hypnotics, tranquilizers)	Short acting (hypnotics)
Chlordiazepoxide	Alprazolam	Midazolam
Clorazepate	Flunitrazepam	Triazolam
Clobazam	Lorazepam	
Diazepam	Nitrazepam	
	Oxazepam	
	Temazepam	

Note. Main uses are indicated in parentheses.

Side effects of benzodiazepines include seizures and a return of acute anxiety on rapid withdrawal, concentration and memory impairment, ataxia, and fetal hypotonia. The inverse agonists are both proconvulsant and anxiogenic.

Benzodiazepines differ with regard to duration of action (see Table 14–4). Several are used to control epilepsy, most often in patients with *status epilepticus*. The main ones used in oral therapy of epilepsy are clobazam and clonazepam. Benzodiazepines are also used as hypnotics, to treat spasticity and myoclonus, and to induce preoperative amnesia. Clonazepam has been given in large doses in patients with acute mania.

Buspirone is an azaspirodecanedione, nonbenzodiazepine anxiolytic that is a 5-HT$_{1a}$ agonist. It does not show cross-tolerance with the benzodiazepines and has fewer sedative and amnestic effects. Its main disadvantage is its delayed onset of action, which may be up to 2 weeks.

■ MOOD-STABILIZING DRUGS

Lithium is used to stabilize mood, and its mode of action is unknown. It is used in a number of cyclical conditions, such as bipolar affective disorder, recurrent affective disorder, cluster headache, migraine, and paroxysmal aggression. It has a number of side effects (see Table 14–5).

Side effects of lithium can be avoided to some extent by monitoring serum lithium levels; treatment with lithium is one of the main indications for routine monitoring of serum levels of psychotropic drugs. Severe intoxication may lead to a delirium and subsequent encephalopathy. Severe central nervous system (CNS) side effects are occasionally seen at lithium levels below the given upper limits of tolerance.

TABLE 14–5. **Side effects of lithium**

Neuropsychiatric	**Gastrointestinal**
Drowsiness	Anorexia, nausea, vomiting
Confusion, stupor	Diarrhea
Psychomotor retardation	Dry mouth
Restlessness	Weight gain
Headache	**Renal**
Muscle weakness	Microtubular lesions
Tremor	Polyuria
Ataxia	**Cardiovascular**
Myasthenia gravis–like syndrome	Hypotension
	Electrocardiogram changes
Peripheral neuropathy	**Endocrine**
Choreoathetoid movements	Myxedema
Dysarthria	Thyrotoxicosis
Dysgeusia	Hyperparathyroidism
Blurred vision	**Other**
Seizures	Polydipsia
Dizziness	Glycosuria
Vertigo	Hypercalcuria
	Rashes

■ ANTICONVULSANT DRUGS

It has become fashionable to refer to anticonvulsant drugs as antiepileptic drugs. Although they have antiseizure activity, they also have a range of other activities including important psychotropic actions. Carbamazepine and valproate have antimanic and mood-stabilizing properties; carbamazepine is used in *trigeminal neuralgia*, paroxysmal aggressive disorders, and schizophrenia.

Recently, several new drugs have been introduced, including vigabatrin (a suicidal inhibitor of GABA-transaminase that elevates CNS GABA), felbamate, lamotrigine, and gabapentin.

The suggested sites of action of anticonvulsants are shown in Table 14–6. The half-life, recommended serum levels, and some other properties are shown in Table 14–7. The indications for use of these agents are shown in Figure 14–2.

Serum level monitoring is especially important for phenytoin. This drug has nonlinear pharmacokinetics (Figure 14–3) and interacts with several other drugs (Table 14–8). Drugs that induce the liver cytochrome P_{450} system—oxidative enzymes most involved

TABLE 14–6. **Suggested sites of action of anticonvulsants**

Drug	GABA receptor	Channel gNa	gCaT
Phenytoin	−	++	−
Carbamazepine	−	++	?
Valproic acid	+/?	+	−
Phenobarbitone	+	+	−
Clonazepam	++	+	−
Clobazam	++	?	−
Ethosuximide	−	−	+
Vigabatrin	++	?	−

Note. ++, +, and − indicate approximate strength of effects.
GABA = γ-aminobutyric acid. gCaT = T-calcium current conductance.
gNa = sodium conductance.

TABLE 14–7. **Some clinical properties of anticonvulsants**

Drug	Half-life (h)	Recommended serum level (μmol/L[a])	Indications
Carbamazepine	8–45	16–50	Generalized seizures; simple or complex partial seizures; secondary generalized seizures
Clobazam	22	. . .	As for carbamazepine, plus generalized absence and myoclonic seizures
Clonazepam	20–40	. . .	Myoclonic seizures
Ethosuximide	30–100	300–700	Generalized absence of seizures
Gabapentin	5–7	. . .	Refractory partial and generalized seizures
Lamotrigine	20–30	. . .	Refractory partial and generalized seizures
Phenobarbitone (children)	36	60–180	Generalized simple seizures or complex partial seizures
Phenytoin	9–140	40–100	Generalized seizures; simple or complex partial seizures
Primidone	3–12	. . .	Generalized: complex or simple partial seizures
Sodium valproate	10–15	350–700	Generalized absence seizures; myoclonic seizures; simple or complex partial seizures
Vigabatrin	5–7	. . .	Partial and secondary generalized seizures

Note. For conversion of μmol/L to μg/ml, divide by the number indicated: carbamazepine, 4; ethosuximide, 7; phenobarbitone, 4; phenytoin, 4; sodium valproate, 7.

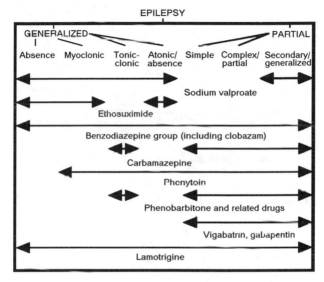

FIGURE 14–2. Spectrum of anticonvulsant activity.

in the breakdown of anticonvulsants—lower the levels of drugs that also use the liver for metabolism. Carbamazepine induces its own hepatic metabolism, with serum levels falling despite a constant dosage in the first weeks of therapy. Metabolism of lamotrigine is inhibited by valproate, and patients on the latter require lower starting doses and smaller increases in dose of lamotrigine. Vigabatrin and gabapentin seem devoid of significant interactions with other anticonvulsants.

The side effects of anticonvulsant drugs are shown in Table 14–9. Of special neuropsychiatric interest are cognitive impairment and movement disorders with phenytoin, encephalopathy and tremor with valproate, psychosis and depression with vigabatrin, depression with phenobarbitone, and acute dystonia with car-

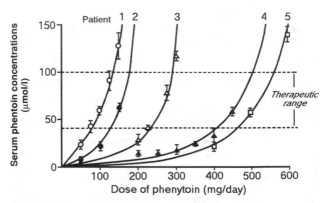

FIGURE 14–3. Nonlinear metabolism of phenytoin in three patients.

bamazepine. In some cases, especially the psychoses, these effects are seen with suppression of seizures (see discussion of forced normalization in Chapter 8). Although agranulocytosis has been associated with carbamazepine, it is very rare and can occur with several other anticonvulsants; it is not necessary to continually monitor hematological indices in patients receiving it. Patients should notify their physicians immediately if petechiae, pallor, weakness, fever, or infection occurs.

Use of felbamate has been severely restricted after reports of cases of aplastic anemia.

■ ABREACTION

With abreaction, the patient is encouraged to relax and reveal emotional conflicts to the examiner. Catharsis is one aim. Abreaction can be an aid to diagnosis (e.g., in cases of stupor) and an effective treatment in conversion disorders. It can be achieved with hypnosis or with slow intravenous injection of a drug such as Amytal sodium or diazepam in the presence of an anesthesiologist

TABLE 14–8. **Significant anticonvulsant interactions**

Interaction	Drug
Anticonvulsants that reduce phenytoin levels	Diazepam, clonazepam, carbamazepine,[a] phenobarbitone, vigabatrin[b]
Anticonvulsants that increase free phenytoin levels	Valproate[c]
Other drugs whose effect is reduced by anticonvulsants (by increased hepatic metabolism)	Warfarin and coumarin anticoagulants, cortisol, dexamethasone, prednisolone, oral contraceptives, vitamin D, phenylbutazone, antidepressants, chlorpromazine, digoxin, diazepam
Other drugs that may induce anticonvulsant toxicity	Isoniazid, dicumarol, disulfiram, chloramphenicol, imipramine, chlorpromazine, chlorpheniramine, methylphenidate, erythromycin

[a]Carbamazepine reduces the serum concentration of phenytoin and vice versa.
[b]Not clinically significant, mechanism unknown.
[c]Sodium valproate displaces phenytoin from its protein-binding sites, increasing the unbound fraction of phenytoin.

in case of respiratory arrest. Patients are informed the injection will make them relaxed and drowsy and allow them to talk about conflictual issues.

■ ELECTROCONVULSIVE THERAPY

The mode of action of ECT is unknown, although von Meduna introduced convulsive therapy after observations of an antagonism between psychotic symptoms and seizures in some epileptic patients. The concept of *forced normalization* (see Chapter 8) may be relevant to understanding its mode of action.

There is no convincing evidence that waveform (sine wave or brief-pulse stimuli) affects outcome, although low-energy stimuli

TABLE 14–9.   **Side effects of anticonvulsants**

Nervous system	**Skin**
Cerebellar atrophy	Hirsutism
Peripheral neuropathy	Pigmentation
Encephalopathy	Acne
Psychoses, depression	Rashes
Hematopoietic system	Alopecia
Folic acid deficiency	**Endocrine system**
Neonatal coagulation defects	Pituitary-adrenal
Agranulocytosis	Thyroid-parathyroid
Skeletal systems	Hyperglycemia (diabetogenic)
Metabolic bone disease	**Other metabolic disorders**.
Vitamin D deficiency	Vitamin B_6 deficiency (?)
Connective tissue	Heavy metals
Gum hypertrophy	**Immunologic disorders**
Facial skin changes	Lymphotoxicity
Wound healing	Lymphadenopathy
Dupuytren's contracture	Systemic lupus erythematosus
Liver	Antinuclear antibodies
Enzyme induction	Immunoglobulin changes (?)
Hepatotoxicity	Immunosuppression

evoke fewer cognitive and electrophysiologic abnormalities. The seizure is crucial to the observed clinical effects on behavior. These effects differ depending on the clinical syndrome being treated (Table 14–10).

Unilateral electrode placement is slightly less effective than bilateral electrode placement; however, unilateral electrode placement is associated with fewer complaints of postseizure confusion, memory disruption, and headache.

The main indication for ECT is mood disorder, especially delusional depressive states. ECT has been shown to be helpful in some cases of schizophrenia, catatonia, neurologic disorders associated with severe depression, delirium, mania, Parkinson's disease, and epilepsia partialis continua.

TABLE 14–10. **Effects of electroconvulsive therapy in different clinical syndromes**

Clinical syndrome	Effect
Major depression	Relief of depression
Psychosis	Normalized thought patterns
Excitement, mania	Reduced motility
Stupor	Increased alertness
Parkinsonism	Reduced rigidity
Pseudodementia	Relief of dementia
Neuroleptic malignant syndrome	Syndrome relief
Hypochondriasis	Worse symptoms
Hysterical character	Increased complaints
Denial personality	Increased denial

Contraindications are few but include a recent cerebrovascular accident and the presence of an intracranial tumor. ECT is best avoided when raised intracranial pressure is suspected.

■ NEUROSURGICAL PROCEDURES

Early neurosurgical operations involved destruction of large tracts of white matter to and from the frontal lobes. The current more refined procedures are shown in Table 14–11. Stereotactic procedures allow for greater accuracy and the placement of smaller lesions.

TABLE 14–11. **Neurosurgical procedures for psychiatric illness**

Operation	Targets
Orbital undercutting	Medial frontothalamic fibers
Cingulotomy	Bilateral cingulum
Subcaudate tractotomy	Head of caudate nucleus
Capsulotomy	Internal capsule
Amygdalotomy	Medial amygdala

The main pathways severed pass from the lower medial quadrant of the frontal lobes to the septal and nucleus accumbens areas, the thalamus, and the hypothalamus. Additional target areas are frontocingular and frontohippocampal projections.

The main indications are severe obsessive-compulsive disorder, severe anxiety states, and severe depression. Patients must have been ill for several years, be potentially suicidal, and have failed to respond to alternative therapies. Patients from stable backgrounds with good premorbid personalities do best. Sociopathy is a contraindication, and patients addicted to drugs and alcohol are not suitable. The main complications are cerebral hemorrhage, seizures, suicide, incontinence, weight gain, sleep disturbance, personality changes, and diabetes insipidus.

■ REFERENCES AND RECOMMENDED READING

Altamura AC, Montgomery SA: Fluoxetine dose, pharmacokinetics and clinical efficiency. Reviews in Contemporary Pharmacotherapy 1:75–81, 1990

Bridges P: Psychosurgery revisited. J Neuropsychiatry Clin Neurosci 2:326–331, 1990

Crow TJ, Johnson EC: Controlled trials of ECT. Ann N Y Acad Sci 462:12–29, 1986

Fink M: Convulsive therapy and epilepsy research, in What Is Epilepsy? Edited by Trimble MR, Reynolds EH. Edinburgh, Scotland, Churchill Livingstone, 1986, pp 217–228

Lieberman JA: Understanding the mechanism of action of atypical antipsychotic drugs. Br J Psychiatry 163 (suppl 22):7–18, 1993

Post RM, Trimble MR, Pippinger C: Clinical Use of Anticonvulsants in Psychiatric Disorders. New York, Demos, 1989

Richelson E: The newer antidepressants, structures, pharmacokinetics, pharmacodynamics and proposed mechanism of action. Psychopharmacol Bull 20:313–323, 1986

Trimble MR (ed): New Anticonvulsant Drugs. Chichester, England, Wiley, 1994

Trimble MR: Biological Psychiatry, 2nd Edition. Chichester, England, Wiley, 1996

GLOSSARY

Affect The outward expression of emotion—for example, the facial expressions associated with sadness or happiness. Mood and affect are usually congruent but may become dissociated in neurologic disorders (e.g., pseudobulbar palsy and specific types of epilepsy) that produce changes in affect without corresponding alterations in mood.

Abreaction The procedure of reviving to consciousness traumatic or forgotten experiences, usually associated with the expression of pent-up emotion.

Acalculia The inability to calculate accurately. Visuospatial acalculia, aphasia-related acalculia, and primary anarithmetrias are recognized.

Achromatopsia Acquired color blindness.

Agnosia The inability to recognize an object despite intact perception and adequate cognition. The precept is stripped of its meaning.

Agraphia The acquired inability to write. Mechanical and aphasic agraphias are known.

Akathisia A strong, unpleasant subjective sense of the need to move manifested by restless and fidgety movements.

Akinesia Poverty of movement.

Alexia The acquired inability to read. Alexia without agraphia, alexia with agraphia, and a frontal alexia occur clinically.

Anarithmetria A primary acalculia in which the patient has lost the ability to calculate; the disability is not attributable to visuospatial or linguistic deficits.

Aneurysm An abnormal localized dilation of an arterial lumen. In true aneurysms, the vessel intima herniates through the muscularis of the normal arterial wall.

Angular gyrus syndrome The syndrome occurring with dysfunction of the left angular gyrus and characterized by agraphia, alexia, acalculia, right-left disorientation, finger agnosia, right-left disorientation, apraxia, anomia, and verbal amnesia.

Anosognosia Denial of hemiparesis.

Anton's syndrome A syndrome characterized by blindness and denial of the blindness.

Aphasia Loss or impairment of language caused by brain dysfunction.

Apperceptive visual agnosia Clinical syndrome in which the patient can perceive and interpret elementary visual information such as line thickness, line direction, and intensity of shading, but more complex visual stimuli (e.g., letters) cannot be recognized, and the patient cannot draw perceived objects.

Apraxia The inability to follow a command despite normal motor and sensory function and intact comprehension. The individual can typically perform the act spontaneously but not on verbal command (e.g., the individual will spontaneously lick his or her lips but cannot do so when requested by the examiner).

Aprosodia Alteration of the melody and inflection of verbal output.

Associative visual agnosia Clinical syndrome in which the patient can perceive and copy all visual stimuli but cannot interpret them. When the stimulus is presented in another modality (such as touch), the patient immediately recognizes it.

Asterixis Distal flapping-type movement induced by sudden interruption of muscle contraction (negative myoclonus).

Astrocytoma Tumor of astrocytic cells. Four grades of malignancy are recognized: grades 1 and 2 are low-grade, slow-growing tumors; grades 3 and 4 are aggressive tumors called glioblastoma multiforme.

Athetosis Slow, sinuous, writhing movements affecting primarily the distal extremities.

Automatisms Automatic motor acts carried out in a state of altered consciousness.

Balint's syndrome Clinical syndrome characterized by sticky fixation (difficulty interrupting and redirecting gaze), optic ataxia, and simultanagnosia.

Ballismus Uncontrollable, large-amplitude proximal limb movements usually associated with lesions of the subthalamic nucleus.

Bioavailability The proportion of a drug that reaches its site of action after administration.

Bradyphrenia Slowing of mental processes.

Broca's aphasia A nonfluent aphasia with intact comprehension and impaired repetition.

Catatonia Either symptoms of abnormal motor activity, with negativism, autism, or rigidity, or a variety of illness, such as catatonic schizophrenia, in which the outstanding symptoms are motoric.

Catharsis Literally, a purgation, the relief obtained by expression of emotion.

Charcot-Wilbrand syndrome Absence of mental imagery or the capacity for revisualization.

Charles Bonnet syndrome Visual hallucinations associated with ocular pathology in elderly persons.

Chorea Irregular, unpredictable, brief, jerky movements that occur randomly in different body parts.

Cingulum The fiber bundle within the cingulate gyrus that connects frontal and parietal cortex to the parahippocampal gyrus and adjacent medial temporal regions.

Clearance Volume of plasma cleared of a drug in a unit of time.

Cloning The process of producing identical replicas.

Coma   A state of unconsciousness from which a patient cannot be aroused.

Compliance   The ability of a patient to stick to a prescribed regimen of treatment.

Compulsions   Repetitive behaviors (e.g., hand washing, checking the locks, checking to see if the lights have been turned out, repeating what others say) or mental activities (e.g., counting the words in a sentence or other counting activities) that the individual feels compelled to do. Compulsions are typically experienced as involuntary and serving no realistic need of the individual.

Concussion   Immediate and transient impairment of consciousness due to a brain injury.

Confabulation   Detailed description of a past event that is patently false.

Constructional disturbance   Difficulty with copying or drawing figures. Sometimes called "constructional apraxia," but the patients' conditions do not meet common definitions of apraxia.

Contrecoup   Literally, damage at the opposite pole of the brain from the site injured.

Contusion   Damage (to the brain) with injury that does not lead to laceration.

Cortical blindness   Blindness due to bilateral occipital lesions.

Déjà vu   A feeling that an event has been experienced before.

Delirium   Abnormal mental state characterized by the inability to maintain, shift, or properly focus attention. Usually due to a toxic or metabolic disturbance affecting brain function.

Delusion   A false belief based on an incorrect inference about reality. The belief is not part of the person's culture or religion.

Dementia of depression   Dementia syndrome produced by a depressive mood disorder.

Dementia   Syndrome of acquired intellectual impairment affecting memory and at least two cognitive domains and producing social or occupational impairment. Delirium is absent.

Demyelination   The process of destruction of myelin by disease.

Depersonalization   A sense of detachment from oneself. The individual may have the experience of seeing himself or herself from outside as if he or she were an observer.

Derealization   A sense of detachment from the world, as if one is in a dream.

Dysarthria   Disturbance of the mechanical production of speech; abnormal speech articulation.

Dyskinesia   An alternate term for hyperkinesia, usually not including tremors.

Dysmyelination   Abnormal development of myelin.

Dystonia   Spasmodic or sustained postures produced by abnormal, involuntary, sustained, patterned, and often repetitive contraction muscles.

Echolalia   Repetition of what others say.

Engram   The changes in the brain that represent stored memory.

Environmental agnosia   The acquired inability to recognize familiar environments despite intact perception.

Ependymoma   Tumor of ependymal cells lining the ventricular system.

Epilepsy   The liability to recurrent seizures.

Eutonia   A sense of well-being often despite the presence of serious or life-threatening illness.

Formal thought disorder   Inability to think abstractly, with failure of causal links in thinking.

Fugue   Episodes of wandering associated with amnesia.

Gerstmann syndrome The syndrome of right-left disorientation, finger agnosia, dysgraphia, and acalculia occurring with lesions of the left angular gyrus.

Glioblastoma Highly malignant astrocytoma (grades 3 and 4).

Half-life of a drug Time taken for the drug's concentration in plasma to fall by 50%.

Hallucination A sensory perception that occurs without stimulation of the appropriate sensory organ. Nonpsychotic individuals are aware of the unreality of the experiences (e.g., visual hallucinations occurring in the course of migraine); the psychotic individual is unaware of the unreality of the perceptions (e.g., auditory hallucinations of people saying critical things as part of a persecutory psychosis).

Hamartoma A congenital lesion of disordered cell differentiation and migration.

Hemorrhage When applied to the brain, this refers to extravasation of blood into the brain tissue (intraparenchymal hemorrhage) or the subarachnoid space (subarachnoid hemorrhage).

Hydrocephalus Abnormally enlarged ventricles.

Illusion Perceptual distortion of an actual experience (e.g., seeing a chair as if it were a seated person).

Inborn error of metabolism Inherited abnormality of enzyme function leading to abnormal accumulation or deposition of metabolites or a deficiency of specific products.

Interictal Occurring between seizures.

Kindling A phenomenon in which repeated subthreshold electrical stimulation leads to the subsequent development of a seizure and a permanent increase in the epileptogenicity of the brain.

Lability Rapidly changing mood or affect. Lability of affect is present in pseudobulbar palsy. Lability of mood is present in patients with lesions of the orbitofrontal cortex.

Lateralization The concept that specific functions of the brain are mediated preferentially by the action of either the right or the left hemisphere.

Learning The process of acquiring new information.

Ligand A substance that binds to a receptor.

Localization The concept that specific functions are exclusively associated with specific areas of the brain.

Logoclonia Repetition of the final syllables of a word ("Episcopal-copal-copal").

Mannerisms Exaggerated components of normal movements.

Memory The ability to register, recall, and recognize learned information.

Meningioma Tumor of meningeal cells, particularly arachnoidal cells.

Metastasis Tumors that develop from cells that originated in a primary tumor elsewhere in the body and were transported to another location (cells are usually transported through the vascular system).

Mood A pervasive emotional state such as sadness, elation, or anger.

Mutism The absence of verbal output.

Myelin The substance that covers axons and gives the brain its white matter.

Myoclonus Rapid, brief, shocklike muscle jerks of sufficient strength to move a body part.

Neglect Tendency to ignore stimuli on one side of the body.

Obsessions Recurrent and intrusive thoughts, images, or impulses that occur involuntarily. The intrusion of violent or sexual thoughts into the stream of consciousness is typical of obsessions.

Palilalia   Repetition of words or phrases just uttered ("I had eggs for breakfast, eggs for breakfast").

Paramnesia   Distortion of memory with inaccuracy of recall.

Parkinsonism   Combination of akinesia and rigidity with or without rest tremor.

Perseveration   The continuation or recurrence of an experience or activity without an appropriate stimulus. Three types of perseveration are recognized: 1) recurrence of a previous response to a subsequent stimulus, 2) inappropriate maintenance of an activity (as seen on the Wisconsin Card Sorting Test), and 3) abnormal continuation or prolongation of an activity without cessation of a current behavior (Figures 4–2 and 4–3). Perseveration may affect motor acts, thoughts, verbal output, and other activities.

Phosphenes   Flashes of light, usually secondary to retinal or optic nerve disease.

Posttraumatic amnesia   The length of time after a head injury that it takes for a continuous stream of consciousness to return and a continuous stream of memories to be laid down.

Prefrontal   The area immediately in front of the premotor cortex in the frontal lobe.

Premotor   The area immediately in front of the motor cortex in the frontal lobe. Area 6 of Brodmann's map.

Prosopagnosia   Inability to recognize familiar faces.

Pseudodementia   Apparent impairment of cognitive function secondary to a psychiatric illness such as depression, mania, or schizophrenia. The patient can often be shown to perform normally under some circumstances.

Psychosis   Delusions are sufficient by themselves to define a psychotic disorder. Many psychoses are also characterized by hallucinations that occur without insight into the false nature of the experience. Psychotic states frequently have additional positive elements such as disorganized speech, derailment of thought, and catatonia.

Reduplicative paramnesia The belief that one is simultaneously in two locations (e.g., in one hospital within another hospital).

Retrograde amnesia The period that cannot be recalled prior to the occurrence of a brain injury producing an amnestic disorder.

Seizure The main symptom of epilepsy. It is a paroxysmal event caused by abnormal electrochemical discharge in the nervous system and is often accompanied by identifiable changes on a simultaneously recorded electroencephalogram.

Simultanagnosia The inability to perceive more than one object at a time.

Status epilepticus Recurrent seizures without a return of consciousness between attacks.

Steady state When the amount (of a drug) absorbed equals the amount eliminated, and plasma concentrations are stable.

Stereotypies Repeated sequences of complex but purposeless movements.

Stroke Sudden onset of a neurologic deficit due to a cerebrovascular event (thrombosis or hemorrhage).

Stuttering Speech abnormality characterized by repetition of the initial or middle phonemes of words ("be-be-be-because") or the prolongation or arrest of speech sounds.

Syndrome A constellation of signs and symptoms that coalesce to form a recognizable entity with definable characteristics.

Tics Repetitive, irregular, stereotyped movements or vocalizations. Simple tics are brief contractions such as a facial twitch; more complex tics may involve coordinated movement such as touching or bowing.

Transcortical motor aphasia Nonfluent aphasia with intact comprehension and intact repetition.

Tremor Involuntary rhythmic oscillating movement usually resulting from alternating or synchronous reciprocally innervated antagonistic muscles.

Vorbeireden The symptom of approximate answers that are given to simple questions.

INDEX

*Page numbers printed in **boldface** type refer to tables or figures.*

242